LIVER-BRAIN RELATIONSHIPS

LIVER-BRAIN RELATIONSHIPS

By

IAN A. BROWN, M.D., Ph.D.

Associate-Professor of Neurology

Division of Neurology

Department of Neurology and Psychiatry

University of Minnesota

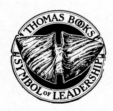

CHARLES C THOMAS · PUBLISHER

Springfield · Illinois · U.S.A.

CHARLES C THOMAS · PUBLISHER
BANNERSTONE HOUSE
301-327 East Lawrence Avenue, Springfield, Illinois, U.S.A.

Published simultaneously in the British Commonwealth of Nations by
BLACKWELL SCIENTIFIC PUBLICATIONS, LTD., OXFORD, ENGLAND

Published simultaneously in Canada by
THE RYERSON PRESS, TORONTO

Library of Congress Catalog Card Number: 57-12538

Printed in the United States of America

To Marian

PREFACE

T HE TITLE of this monograph implies a discussion of the many pertinent and intimate relationships that exist between the liver and the brain and in addition it obviates the necessity of drawing any definitive conclusions. To express any conclusions at all in the preface to a work is a reversal of the usual state of affairs but in this instance justification seems to be satisfied, for the subject of this monograph concerns the relationships that exist between two titanic multifunctioning organs whose normal metabolism is but partially understood. How, then, in the face of this are we able to justify any conclusions concerning causes and treatment of a faulty relationship when we are not completely prepared to assess the normal state of affairs? The liver and the brain would appear to be mutually dependent upon one another to some extent. The former, while it manufactures substances utilized by the brain is indirectly dependent for this function upon the integrity of portions of the brain especially those that regulate respiration and blood flow. The direct dependency of the liver on the function of the brain is not so binding since the former continues to function after severance of its nerve supply. Furthermore, the dependency of brain and liver is not solely a direct one between the two but also operates indirectly through other organs such as the spleen, pancreas, kidneys and adrenals. We are then in no position to draw any conclusions as to the cause of brain dysfunction in hepatic disease in the light of current knowledge. This monograph is but a discussion of the relationships that exist between the organs and no pretense is made to solve the problem.

The material of this monograph was originally presented as a thesis to the University of Minnesota in 1953. The anticipated unravelling of the hepato-cerebral riddle did not materialize between that time and the present. The relationships, theoretical possibilities, causes and effects are re-expressed in the light of recent observations. The clinical studies were done before 1953 and unfortunately tests of ammonia metabolism, urinary amino acid excretion were spotty and therefore lacking in statistical value. Nonetheless such studies as are included here allowed some comparison of liver function during coma and during lesser degree of brain involvement. The clinical case load used in a study of the comatose state also provided the material for the chapter on the pathological aspects.

This monograph includes some historical information which is always a welcome respite to the confining presentation of scientific observations. History, aside from its interest, serves us in other ways too, for it reminds us of our general inadequacies and like the beacon of light behind us it shines on ahead and provides some guidance to the general direction that we should follow. At present we are somewhere in the beam of light but we are nowhere near its end.

The liver itself is discussed in one chapter. To the general practitioner and the specialist of internal medicine this particular portion will have no appeal. It is not included for such individuals but rather it is included for the non-abdominal specialists who are unfamiliar with the organ. For these persons, refreshment of hepatic knowledge is provided, albeit briefly, in the hope that it may aid in a better understanding of the relationships between the liver and the brain.

A chapter of the original thesis on the experimental aspects of this relationship along with some experimental work on cerebral changes in animals with dietary induced liver damage has been omitted. It would seem to this observer that information gained from animal study cannot be effectively applied to the human and this is especially true in assessing the relationship of two organs which exhibit considerable differences between lower and higher forms of life. What is needed more than any other factor is the detection of biochemical changes in human tissues and fluids. Considerable progress has been made along these lines, an example of which is to be seen in the knowledge gained over the past five years in Wilson's disease. The failure to demonstrate positive correlationships between liver pathology and liver function tests for example does not entirely negate the presence of correlative factors but more important it points to the inadequacies of our test parameters. We can only deny correlationships with the tests that were used. That liver function tests and cerebral function tests are of limited application and not the last word is quite obvious to any one in either field who keeps abreast of the literature or who deals with patients.

For assistance, guidance and help in the preparation of this monograph words of appreciation must be extended to several individuals. To Dr. Fae Y. Tichy, formerly Associate Professor of the Division of Neurology of this University, I would like to express my gratitude for her contributions on pathological matters. I am indebted also to Dr. Fred W. Hoffbauer, Associate Professor of the Department of Medicine for his helpful criticisms and contributions, and to Dr. C. J. Watson, Professor and Chairman of the Department of Medicine of the University of Minnesota Hospitals in whose wards the case material was studied. Further appreciation is extended to the librarians of the University Biomedical Library and especially to Mrs. Nollman who was particularly helpful. Words of appreciation are also extended to Mr. Robert Benassi who prepared most of the drawings.

I. A. B.

University of Minnesota

CONTENTS

LIVER-BRAIN RELATIONSHIPS

ENCEPHALO-MYELO BRANCH SYSTEM

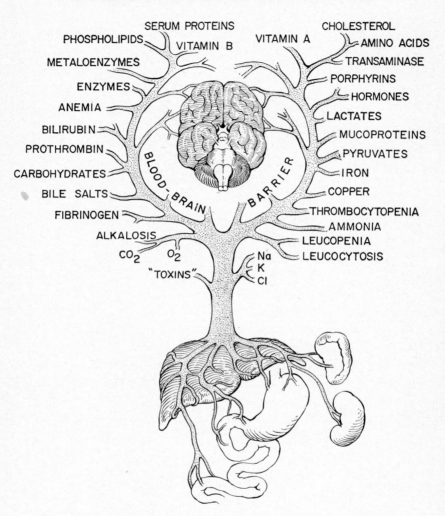

SERUM PROTEINS
PHOSPHOLIPIDS
VITAMIN B
VITAMIN A
CHOLESTEROL
AMINO ACIDS
METALOENZYMES
TRANSAMINASE
ENZYMES
PORPHYRINS
HORMONES
ANEMIA
LACTATES
BILIRUBIN
MUCOPROTEINS
PROTHROMBIN
PYRUVATES
CARBOHYDRATES
IRON
BILE SALTS
COPPER
FIBRINOGEN
THROMBOCYTOPENIA
AMMONIA
ALKALOSIS
LEUCOPENIA
CO_2 O_2 Na   LEUCOCYTOSIS
K
Cl
"TOXINS"

BLOOD-BRAIN   BARRIER

HEPATO-SPLENO-RENAL-INTESTINAL ROOT SYSTEM

Frontispiece: The cerebro-hepatic riddle. The liver-brain relationship can be expressed in a variety of ways. The surrealistic drawing depicts this relationship in the form of a tree. The root system covers more than just the liver. The trunk conveys a multiplicity of abnormal metabolites to the brain. The blood brain barrier is a formidable fortress to be breached before these metabolites reach the brain. Lastly the cerebral blood dynamics bio-physical and bio-chemical reactions must be considered and studied before we can solve this riddle.

Chapter I

HISTORICAL REVIEW

IN ANY historical account concerning matters unsolved or in-completely understood, the question is invariably raised—at what point does history end? Today's discoveries are just as much to-morrow's history as are the discoveries and events of past cen-turies. Where then shall one draw the line between what is historical and what is not? Obviously history is a continuum and justifiably one could include all known facts about the rela-tionship between the liver and the brain under this heading. To do so, however, would be to obscure the historical aspects and substitute completeness and clarity for confusion and brevity. The following historical review of this relationship will span more than twenty centuries although emphasis will be placed on the two most recent—the nineteenth and the twentieth. To focus on the current status of this metabolic entanglement this account will embrace three facets namely—the clinical, the experimental and the theoretical.

The association of mental change with jaundice was well known to the time-honored physicians of antiquity, Hippocrates (1) and Galen(us) (2), both of whom noted and recorded the episodic delirium that ofttimes accompanies jaundice. Hippocrates (460-356 B.C.) attributed liver disease to the humors and to the elabo-ration of yellow bile (choler) and black bile (melanchol(er)y) (Fig. 1). He felt the liver was the seat of love and passion and recognizing its effect on the mind he said "those who are mad on account of phlegm are quiet, but those on account of bile are vociferous, vicious and do not keep quiet." Galen (A.D. 150-199), the "Prince of Physicians," considered the liver to be the source of veins, the elaborator of bile and the seat of the mind (Fig. 2). He believed the blood charged with 'natural spirit' was distributed

3

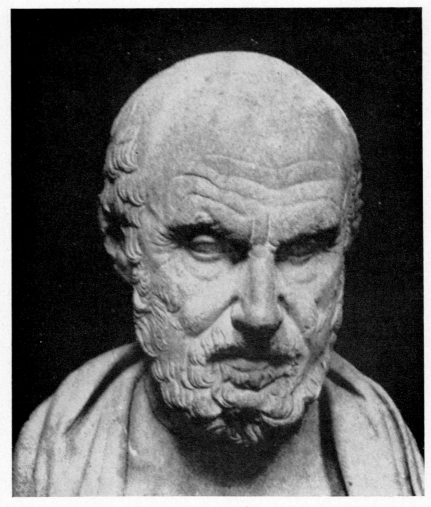

Fig. 1. Hippocrates (c. 460-c. 370 B.C.) Bust in British Museum.
Work of Second or Third Century, B.C.

by the liver and when this reached the heart, it was converted to the 'vital spirit' which bathed the brain (Fig. 3). Galen's contributions to the anatomy of the brain were considerable for he differentiated and named the dura mater, pia mater, corpus collosum, pineal body, pituitary gland, the fornix and seven of the cranial nerves. Despite his many mistakes and apparent fantastic concepts he dominated and obstructed medical thoughts for twelve centuries. The enormous hiatus in medical literature which occurred between the Second and Fourteenth Centuries began to close at the onset of the Renaissance. Mondino (3) (A.D. 1270-1326), a Professor at Bologna, restored anatomy to its rightful place. He felt the liver had 5 lobes (a persistent idea taken from the dogs), and that although yellow bile was secreted by the liver, the black

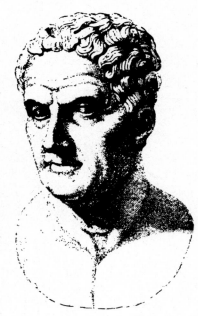

FIG. 2. Claudius Galen (130-201 A.D.). Claudius Galen, a celebrated Greek physician, was born at Pergamos, Mysia. He studied medicine in Alexandria and in other places and was physician to the school of gladiators in his native city for six years. He then went to Rome, where he gained a great reputation, attended the emperor Marcus Aurelius and his two sons, and later, the emperor Severus. Of his works, eighty-three genuine treatises still exist. He gathered all the medical knowledge of his time. His medical work continued to be the authority for centuries. He probably died in Sicily.

bile originated in the spleen and was evacuated through imaginary channels into the cardiac end of the stomach (Fig. 4).

The Renaissance was dominated by artistic endeavours which was reflected in the magnificent anatomical sketches of Leonardo da Vinci (1452-1519) and Andreas Vesalius (1514-1564). With the free thinking and individualism of this period Galen's infallibility was questioned and his anatomical concepts corrected and superceded by those of Vesalius who published in 1543 *De Humani Corporis Fabrica* a magnificent work on anatomy. The medical literature of that era was made primarily by the anatomists and

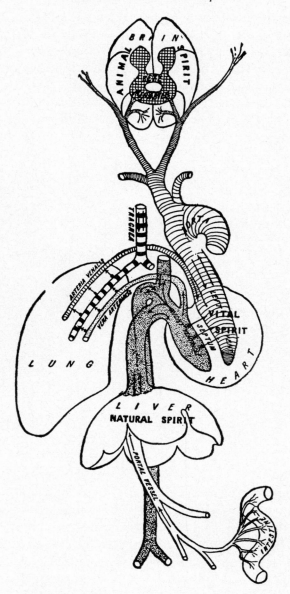

Fig. 3. The Galenic concept of the circulation.

later by clinicians. From the Eighteenth Century onward there has been a voluminous and noteworthy increase in medical literature on the liver and its relationships.

Glissonii (4), a Cambridge Professor of Anatomy, published in 1659 an authoritative and detailed treatise on the anatomy of the

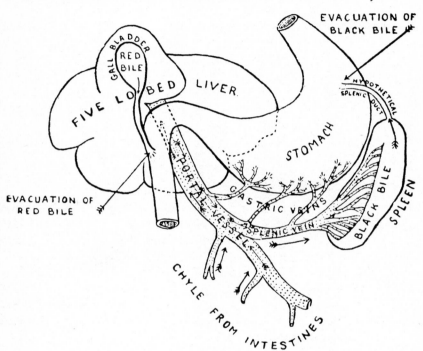

FIG. 4. The mediaeval view of the physiology of the portal system. The portal vessel brings chyle from the intestines to the five lobed liver. Red bile is evacuated from the liver by the bile duct into the duodenum. Blood is sent from the liver to the spleen via the splenic vein. Black bile (melancholy) is evacuated into the stomach either by a hypothetical duct near the cardiac end of the stomach or by the gastric veins.

liver (see Figs. 5 and 6). In addition to leaving his name to the capsule enclosing the liver he looked upon the liver as a peculiar organ for the filtering of bile from the blood (peculaire collatorium) and like many others of his era regarded the bile as the cause of disease in other organs. One year later Rubeous (5) gave the

earliest account of acute yellow atrophy and noted that excitement and coma was often associated with jaundice. A century
later the time honored pathologist, Morgagni (6) in 1761 recorded
the most authentic description of acute yellow atrophy and in
addition to his own observations he cited cases of Baillou, Bonet,

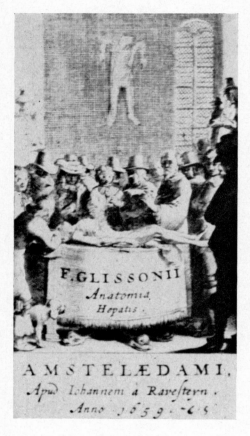

FIG. 5. Photograph from the
Frontispiece of F. Glissoniis text
of 1659. This shows Glissonii,
the tall hatless gesticulating individual to the right of center
demonstrating to his colleagues.

Guarinonius and Valsalva, contemporary authors, all of whom
had observed abnormal mental states including convulsions and
delirium following the onset of jaundice. During the ensuing 75
years little or no literature on this subject appeared. Interest was
revived in 1834 by the appearance of two separate accounts of
hepatic coma in the *London Medical Gazette*. Griffin (7) in one

of these related his experiences with three members of a family with jaundice, two of whom expired in coma. The third, a youth of 11 years, regained consciousness following the application of hot fomentations to the neck, castor oil purgatives and a rather extensive phlebotomy. The success of this therapy was attributed to the castor oil purgation of intestinal toxins. Griffin, in addition, quoted cases of MacLeod who 3 three years previously had briefly described to the Westminster Medical Society of 1832, several

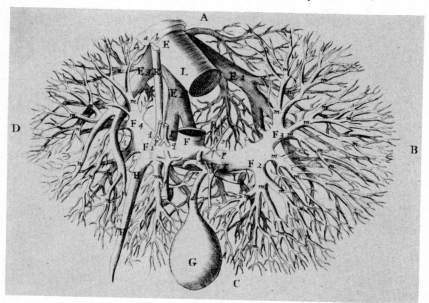

FIG. 6. Cut taken from Glissonii's text of 1659 on the anatomy of the liver.

cases of jaundice which had rapidly terminated in coma following a period of confusion which waxed and waned. Autopsy of one case exhibited only a deep yellow color to the meninges. Aldis (8) in the same publication commented on the absence of cerebral findings at autopsy in the case of a young jaundiced woman who had progressively developed confusion, severe headaches, lethargy and coma.

Bright (9), in 1836, and Budd (10), in 1845, gave excellent accounts of acute fatal jaundice with mental and neurological changes. The former described 8 cases of fatal jaundice of which 5 were autopsied. A case reported by Bright is worthy of mention as it included the features characteristic of hepatic coma as we know them today; namely, dilation of the pupils or pupil, irregular jerking movements of the extremities, dysarthria, flexion of the knees against the abdominal wall, confusion and delirium followed by coma and death. He observed the bile stained cerebral blood vessels and yellow serum from which he reached the conclusion that the neurological symptoms were due to the high concentration of bile in the blood.

The modern approach to the diseases of the liver may well have originated with Frerichs (11), in 1858, when he described in great detail acute yellow atrophy, fatty metamorphosis and cirrhosis of the liver. In an analysis of 31 cases of acute yellow atrophy he noted the similarity of "abnormal conditions of the nervous system" in every case. Furthermore, he distinguished two types of cerebral change, one of excitement and one of depression. The former was characterized by delirium, convulsions, and the latter by progressive lethargy, coma and death. He observed convulsions and noted that in most cases the cerebral alterations appeared simultaneously with the jaundice. In addition, muscular fasciculations, tetany, hiccoughing and dilated pupils were observed. Frerichs commented upon the paucity of pathological changes in the brain at autopsy, a feature which was noted by many others of that era. Up to that time the clinical savants were obsessed with the importance of the bile and blamed disease on its unnatural quantity and color. Frerichs dissented from this view primarily because of a series of experiments in which he injected bile into the veins of dogs without producing any nervous system symptoms. He then expressed his opinion, that the brain derangement was the result of chemical alterations in the blood stream as a consequence of the damaged liver and he stressed hypoglycaemia. The work by Frerichs in three volumes was a masterpiece of its day, being replete with information both clinical and experimental. Used as a text and reference for many years it was subsequently translated and published in New York in 1878.

Schiff (12), in 1877, noted that portal vein ligation was followed by death in a matter of 2 to 3 hours and this was considered to be the consequence of toxins elaborated by the necrotic liver.

In 1883, Westphal (13) published an account in which he observed tremors, dysarthria, slowness of movement and rigidity in 2 patients. Although the patients ultimately died in coma no cerebral changes were noted. Cirrhosis was not mentioned despite the observation that the liver was yellow in color. Because of the clinical resemblance to multiple sclerosis Westphal proposed the term "pseudosclerosis." He did not consider any connection between the neurological findings and the yellow liver.

The term "cholemia" was introduced by Leyden (14), in 1886, because of the resemblance of hepatic coma to the state of uremia. The mental changes were considered to be due to the retention of bile—a view expressed also by Bright (9).

While isolated case reports appeared in the literature describing liver pathology and noting the association of cerebral changes, the first description of a progressive familial disorder associated with liver disease appeared under the title "tetanoid chorea" by Gowers in 1888 (15) and 1906 (16). He described a familial, progressive illness, appearing early in life, in which generalized extensor spasms of the limbs, a fixed vacant facial expression and athetotic movements of the fingers were observed. Post-mortem examination of this case showed no abnormality of the brain grossly or microscopically. Cirrhosis of the liver was not recorded but was mentioned in a later account. In a second case, in 1906, Gowers (16) observed cavitation of the outer layer of the lenticular nucleus on the left. The liver in this case was cirrhotic.

These reports were the forerunners of the entity later described in detail by Kinnier Wilson and known today as hepatolenticular degeneration (Wilson's Disease). A historical review of liver-brain relationships would be quite incomplete without mention, in some detail, of the background and developments that preceded and followed Wilson, since this disorder is the archetype of hepatocerebral relationship (Fig. 7).

Homen, in 1890 (17) and again in 1892 (18), published an account of a disease in which a sister and two brothers in a family of eleven were affected and which was characterized by a hollow,

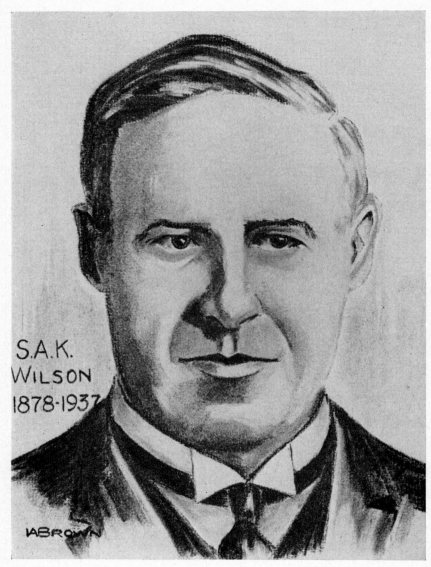

Fig. 7. Samuel Alexander Kinnier Wilson: Born in New Jersey, educated in Edinburgh, studied under Jackson, Dejerine, Bromwell, Gowers and Horsley, his chief contribution was that of his classical paper on Lenticular Degeneration. Wilson was also an excellent teacher.

fatuous facial smile, intention tremor of the hands and legs, marked rigidity of the limbs, drooling of saliva, clonic and tonic muscle spasms and dysphagia. Post-mortem examination showed bilateral cavitation of the lenticular nucleus and an advanced degree of cirrhosis of the liver. The relation of the cirrhosis to the degeneration of the lenticular nucleus, however, was not mentioned.

Ormerod (19) in 1890 published a third case characterized by signs of involvement of the extrapyramidal system, fever, delirium, and an advanced degree of cirrhosis of the liver. Autopsy demonstrated bilateral softening of the putamen. No microscopic changes were noted. Both Ormerod and Gowers were impressed by the occasional variation in the symptoms and pointed out that a diagnosis of hysteria could have been made with reason by virtue of the curious disproportion of the clinical appearance and the actual objective signs of an organic involvement of the nervous system. Ormerod for the first time stressed the relationship of the liver cirrhosis to the cerebral changes.

At this time two papers were published in the German literature both of which were to provoke considerable controversy in the elucidation of cerebro-hepatic relationships. One was the introduction of the term and description of the disease, hemochromatosis, by von Recklinghausen (20) in 1889. Of more importance was the revival of the term "pseudosclerosis" by Strümpell (21) in 1898. At this time he described a case showing cirrhosis of the liver associated with tremors, labored speech, rigidity and slow movements. There was no mention of a familial incidence and little importance was attached to the liver pathology. While no cerebral pathology could be demonstrated, Strümpell was convinced the case was organic rather than hysterical, the latter term coming into its own at this time.

Fleischer, in 1909 (22) and in 1912 (23), published reports on the appearance of a golden brown pigmentated ring around the cornea in three cases of pseudosclerosis. Kayser (24), in 1902, had originally described the corneal pigmentation but thought his patient had multiple sclerosis. Anton (25), in 1908, described the case of a young girl of 14 who developed ataxia, choreiform movements, dysarthric speech, hyperreflexia, and focal convulsions. She became completely demented and died of heart failure. Autopsy showed a large area of softening in the frontal lobe and bilateral cavitation of the putamen. The liver was cirrhotic. Although glycosuria was present the condition was felt to be due to congenital cerebral syphilis.

It remained for Wilson (26), in 1912, to tie the loose threads together into one disorder which he called progressive lenticular degeneration. Wilson in a masterful thesis for which he received a gold medal, reviewed the 8 cases reported by Gowers, Homen and Ormerod and added 4 more which he had observed personally. The disease which bears his name was described as a progressive familial condition characterized by cirrhosis of the liver and by generalized tremors, muscle rigidity, muscle spasms, contractures, dysarthria, dysphagia, emaciation and transient psychotic states. Pathologically, he described bilateral softening of the lenticular nucleus and a coarse nodular cirrhosis of the liver. Wilson emphasized the pure striatal symptomatology and the lack of signs of liver dysfunction during life in view of the marked liver pathology evident at autopsy.

Although cognizant of the previous publications of Westphal (13), Strümpell (21) and Fleischer (23), Wilson paid little attention to pseudosclerosis. In an addendum to his thesis on progressive lenticular degeneration he recognized that a close analogy existed and that further study was necessary. He commented upon the incomplete post mortem examinations and the lack of pathological change. He believed, however, that the case of Fleischer (23) belonged in the same category as progressive lenticular degeneration for in his textbook he commented that "the features once imagined to distinguish pseudosclerosis are now valueless and that there is more valid reason to include cases having cirrhotic lesions of the liver under the classification of lenticular degeneration" (27). Potts and Spiller (28), in 1905, like Westphal considered the disorder a variation of multiple sclerosis. Wilson regarded these case reports as so heterogeneous as to be unclassifiable. In a somewhat acid expression of his opinion he stated that the "summary of facts warrants the conclusion that the pseudosclerosis of Westphal-Strümpell not merely violates the canons of nosology but has nothing whatever to do with liver disease." Greenfield, Poynton and Walsh (29) supported this view.

Despite this, the term pseudosclerosis continued to appear in the literature and was used particularly by German authors. Denny-Brown (30) stated that the tremor without postural change, onset later in life and the prolonged course served to separate pseudosclerosis from Wilson's degeneration. However, the real distinguishing feature was considered to be the presence of a remarkable alteration of the cerebral astrocytes first reported by Hösslin and Alzheimer (31) in 1912 and later confirmed by Luthy (32). Campbell and Morse (33), in 1924 believed that the toxins formed as a result of liver damage acted either on the glial or on the neurones. The presence of Alzheimer cells indicated the predominance of glial reaction and the condition was that of pseudosclerosis. On the other hand, if the neuronal changes were the outstanding feature then the condition was that of Wilson's disease. A transitional case showing both degeneration of the lenticular nucleus and widespread distribution of Alzheimer cells was reported by Hall (34) in 1921, and served to bridge the chasm between the two conditions. Hall, in an excellent review, proposed the term hepato-lenticular degeneration. Barnes and Hurst (35, 36), in 1926 and 1929 also reported Alzheimer cells in two cases of Wilson's disease, although in two other members of the same family such cells were not found. Spielmeyer (37) in 1920 observed Alzheimer cells in one case of Wilson's disease. With few exceptions most authorities regarded pseudosclerosis and Wilson's degeneration as variations of one and the same disease.

Pollack (38), in 1917, described corneal pigmentation in the progressive lenticular degeneration of Wilson and commented on its appearance before the development of cerebral changes in some cases. In 1933, Wilson himself described the presence of a corneal ring in a boy of 14 who had other features of progressive lenticular degeneration. Although convinced that the Kayser-Fleischer corneal ring was part of the symptom complex of hepato-lenticular degeneration Wilson stressed that it was not a constant feature.

Variations in the clinical picture of hepato-lenticular degeneration appeared in the literature. In 1916 Bramwell (39) and Kehrer (40), in 1926 reported on the "formes frustes" which Wilson correctly pointed out should only be considered in the presence of symptoms of hepato-lenticular degeneration in other members of the family. Liver symptomatology preceding the onset of cerebral symptoms was reported by Jendralski (41), Kraupa (42), Hadfield (43), and Barnes and Hurst (36). Although Wilson stressed the lack of liver symptomatology during life, two of his published cases had attacks of jaundice preceding the onset of cerebral symptoms. Publication of a case by Borberg (44), in 1927, and by Babonniex and Widiez (45) in the same year showing striatal symptomatology resulting from carcinoma and adenoma of the liver respectively served to bridge the gap between the liver and the brain but did not clarify the Wilsonian aspect of this relationship.

Hemochromatosis was first related to Wilson's disease by Lowy (46), in 1922, when he reported on a brown pigment on the face, neck, axilla and genitalia in a case of hepato-lenticular degeneration. Brouwer (47), in 1936, reported on a case having signs of hepato-lenticular degeneration and hemochromatosis. The patient, a male of 59 years had diabetes, cirrhosis and a bronzed skin. He developed muscular rigidity, a labored gait, dysarthria, dysphagia and increased emotionality. Autopsy confirmed the evidence of hemochromatosis, and the brain showed bilateral cavitation of the caudate nucleus and putamen in addition to scattered Alzheimer cells. Waggoner and Malamud (48) also described a case of hemochromatosis with cerebral symptoms consisting of mental confusion, ataxia, hypertonia, facial palsy, and dysarthria. At autopsy lesions were found in the cortex, putamen, globus pallidus, cerebral peduncles and cerebellar white matter. Thaddea and Oettel (49), in 1940, in a paper entitled "Hemochromatose der Haut bei Morbus Wilson" demonstrated hemosiderin in the skin of a patient with Wilson's disease. Lewey and Goven (50), in 1942, reviewed the literature and added a case of hemochromatosis which they endeavoured to relate to Wilson's disease. Neuman (51), in 1948, McDougal and Adams (52), in 1950, described the neuropathological changes in hemochromatosis. In the latter report 10 of 29 cases expired in hepatic coma. Recent reports by Glazebrook (53), in 1945, and Cumings, in 1948 (54) and 1951 (55), showing an increase in the copper content of brain and liver in hepato-lenticular degeneration and of increased copper content of the liver in hemochromatosis by Sheldon (56) suggests a chemical relationship between the two disorders.

Wilson's paper in 1912 marked a milestone in hepato-cerebral relationships. Here was a condition in which cerebral symptoms appeared first and foremost in contrast to hepatic coma which was the terminal point of pre-existing hepatic disease and subsequent hepatic failure. The striatal symptomatology which Wilson characterized by "involuntary movements, usually of the nature of a tremor, dysarthria, dysphagia, muscular weakness, spasticity and contractures with progressive emaciation; with these there may be associated emotionalism . . . ," was observed as part of the cerebral symptomatology of hepatic insufficiency regardless of the cause. It became apparent to many investigators that the striatal symptom complex in liver disorders was not restricted to Wilson's disease, nor, on the other hand, was Wilson's disease restricted to the striatum.

The controversy that followed in the wake of Wilson's paper, and which centered around the relationships of this disease to pseudosclerosis and hemochromatosis, and which in addition enlarged the disease beyond that described by its architect served to further expand the relationship of these two organs. In passing it is interesting to note that little or no mention of hepatic coma or even recognition of cerebral involvement in liver disease appears in any of the standard texts on the nervous system during the nineteenth century.

Although Wilson's paper dramatically focused attention on the liver-brain complex as no other paper has done before or since two other facets of this relationship continued quietly on without fanfare—namely clinical and experimental investigation of hepatic disease and especially of hepatic coma. Rolleston (57), in 1912, first described the extensor toe response in hepatic coma and this was later confirmed by Wilcox (58) and Elliott and Walshe (59) who observed this phenomenon in hepatic insufficiency due to acute yellow atrophy, cirrhosis and carcinoma of the liver. Adams (60), in 1949, emphasized forced grasping and Walshe (61) in a study noted flexion of the legs upon the abdomen in cases of hepatic coma. Clinical studies of the neurological involvement in hepatic disease without coma appeared with reports by Lucke (62), in 1944, and Stokes, Owen and Hohnes (63), in 1945, as the most noteworthy. Mental changes of a wide variety were reported in hepatolenticular degeneration by Gysin and Cooke (64) and in hepatitis by Leibowitz and Gorman (65). While spinal cord involvement is rare in hepatic disease several case reports by Hardy and Feemster (66), Byrne and Taylor (67) and Lescher (68) attest to its affliction in some instances. Such additional features served to broaden the brain-liver relationship from a narrow concept of advanced hepatic failure with coma, and basal ganglionic degeneration as in Wilson's disease, to one of widespread nervous system involvement with milder degrees of hepatic disease.

The development of electroencephalography in 1927 by Berger and its subsequent application to clinical problems was applied to the elucidation of this relationship. This has been both unrewarding and disappointing.

The experimental approach to this entanglement lagged somewhat behind the clinical studies. The previously mentioned and persistent theory that an abnormality of bile constituted the "agent provocateur" for all the symptoms in hepatic failure prompted Frerichs in 1858 to inject bile into the veins of dogs to determine its effect on the nervous system and while he was able to convince himself that bile was ineffectual, Kuhne (69), who carried out similar experimentation at the same time, was not convinced. The experimental approach to the problem has centered on the production of liver damage either by chemical or surgical means and by procedures designed to exclude the liver from its normal circulatory relationships. Thus the portocaval anastomosis or Eck fistula, ligation of the common bile duct alone or in combination have been devised. The Eck fistula was first applied to this problem by Stolnikow (70). Hahn, Massen, Nencki and Pawlow (71), in 1893, combined the portocaval anastomosis with ligation of the hepatic artery. The syndrome of "meat intoxication" arose as a result of this and similar studies by Fuchs (72), in 1921, Pollack (38), in 1922, Balo and Korpassy (73), in 1932, Bollman and Mann, (74) in 1936, and De Jong (75), in 1945, all of whom observed cerebral changes in Eck fistulized animals in a high protein intake. Hepatic artery ligation was carefully studied by Rappoport (70) and Markovitz, Rappoport and Scott (76), in 1948, Frazer *et al.* (77), in 1951, and Grindlay, Mann and Bollman (78), in 1951. Although the hepatic artery ligation was performed successfully before this time the mortality was high and the survival period too short to allow for the development of symptoms. The advent of penicillin diminished this drawback and made the study of this technique possible. Much of the physiology of the liver was worked out by the technique of hepatectomy. The cerebral effects of ligation of the common bile duct was studied by De Jong (75), in 1945, and Crandall and Weil (79) and others.

Wilson's publication in 1912 stimulated considerable research on liver-brain relationships and was principally directed towards the production of hepatic injury by chemical means. In 1919, Edsall and Drinker (80) and Mella (81), in 1924, used manganese to produce liver damage in animals and which also developed striatal symptomatology and when autopsied were shown to have changes identical with that seen in hepatolenticular degeneration. Chloroform and phosphorus were used in studies by Williamson and Mann in 1923 (82). Mallory (83), in 1925, produced necrosis, cirrhosis and pigmentation of the liver in rabbits exposed to copper. Toxic substances as carbon-tetrachloride, chloroform, phosphorus, arsenic, selenium, manganese, tar, and lead have been employed to produce liver damage. Such studies, however, were directed towards the development of the liver pathology and other than the mention of gross neurological symptoms, no detailed studies have been made on the central nervous system, except by Hurst and Hurst (84).

Dietary means have recently been employed in the production of liver injury with remarkable success. With the use of choline deficient diets and necrogenic yeast diets liver injury can be produced in nearly one hundred per cent of the animals (85). Gyorgy

(86), Himsworth and Glynn (87) and Hartroft (88) have demonstrated the ease of producing fatty, necrotic, and fibrotic livers.

What might be termed the metabolic approach to this relationship had its beginnings in the work of Chesney, Marshall and Rowntree (89), in 1914, who observed elevation of amino acids in cases of hepatic insufficiency. Stadie and Van Slyke (90), in 1920, showed an increase in the excretion of ammonia and titratable amino acids in terminal hepatic coma secondary to acute yellow atrophy. Early investigators were blocked in the evaluation of amino acid metabolism because of the technical difficulties involved but with the re-application of paper chromatography to medicine, the identification of amino acids was made easy. Because of this, Uzman and Brown (91), in 1948, Dent and Walshe (92), in 1949, De Verdier (93), in 1950, and Cooper, Eckhardt, Faloon and Davidson (94), in the same year, have reported changes in the amino acid metabolism in Wilson's disease. Roman (95), in 1927, and Walshe (61), in 1951, have demonstrated an abnormal urinary excretion pattern of amino acids in hepatic coma regardless of the underlying liver pathology. Quastel (96), in 1935, Weil and Malherbe (97), in 1936, studied glutamic acid metabolism in the brain and liver. Walshe (61) demonstrated an increase in glutamine in the spinal fluid cases of hepatic coma and Amatuzio and Nesbitt (98), in 1950, and Snell and Butt (99), in 1941, observed changes in the pyruvic and lactic acid concentrations in the blood in hepatic coma.

Many theories have been advanced over the years in vain attempts to explain the complexities and mysteries of liver-brain relationships. Mention of these is both of historical interest and quite enlightening not only because of the diversity and number of theories evolved but also because some, upon which doubt had been cast in the past, are in the process of revival. Of greater importance is the plain fact that none have ever been proven! The theory with most adherents is nearly 100 years old and has yet to be proven! Perhaps this is what engenders the challenge. This clearly points to the inadequacy of our knowledge and the necessity for more informative instruments. We have reached the point where light microscopy clinical studies and electroencephalography must be substituted and supplemented by newer procedures. The future path is obvious.

In general theories revolved around the cause of hepato-lenticular degeneration and of hepatic coma. In both instances there was further theorizing as to which organ was the primary seat of disease—the liver or the brain. The earliest theoreticians on this matter regarded the bile as the etiological agent of hepatic disease. Despite the work of Frerichs (11) to the contrary, the French continued in this belief. The "toxic" theory was borne at this time and soon investigators were aligned on opposite sides. The issues were, whether or not the liver elaborated a toxin or was unable to "detoxify" substances elaborated in the intestine. While the main discussion raged over the toxic theory two widely divergent theories were advanced neither of which was accepted and both soon dismissed. One was by Budd (10), in 1845, who suggested that jaundice was "consequent to mental distress and was probably caused by it." The other was a theory advanced by Planer (100), in 1854, that cerebral symptoms were due to pigmentary occlusion of the cerebral vessels.

The toxic theory was interwoven with the question as to which organ was the seat of the primary disorder. One side of the question as to whether the brain or the liver was the seat of the primary disorder was upheld by Boenheim (101), in 1920, Nayrac (102), in 1924, and Oberling and Kalbo (103) all of whom regarded the "vegetative centers" or central ganglia of the brain as the primary cause and the liver dysfunction as secondary. Nayrac (102) observed changes in the tubular and infundibular regions of the hypothalamus and considered the liver circulation was disturbed as a result. This theory has few adherents today as there is generalized agreement that the liver disease occurs first.

Most discussants of hepato-lenticular degeneration and of hepatic coma regard the cerebral changes as occurring secondary to the liver damage. A blood borne toxin elaborated by the damaged liver was postulated to account for the cerebral abnormalities. Such a toxic theory was the earliest developed, and has had the most adherents. By the same token it has created the most controversy which has centered around the question as to whether the liver elaborates the toxin itself or whether it fails to detoxify substances reaching it from the intestine. Pollack (38), Lucks (62), Crandall and Weil (79), Croftan (104), Stokes, Owen and Hohnes (63), Baker (105), Adams (60), Leigh and Card (106) believed that the liver failed to detoxify substances from the intestines which therefore reached the central nervous system. In support of this is the experimental work of De Jong (75), Balo and Korpassy (73) both of whom have produced cerebral lesions in dogs following a porto-caval anastomosis and a high meat diet. The demonstration by Crandall and Weil of changes in the rat spinal cord which has been incubated with the serum from dogs with experimentally produced liver damage lends additional support. More recently Rappoport (70), in 1951, Fraser, Rappoport, Vuylstehe and Colwell (77), in 1951, have prevented the rapid death which follows hepatic artery ligation by the administration of antibiotics thus preventing bacterial toxins from reaching the brain. Against this source of a toxin according to Walshe (61) is the fact that no toxin has ever been isolated nor has it been proved that such a toxin is an abnormal product of digestion or that the intestinal wall is permeable to it. The word "toxin" has been loosely used. There has been no unanimity of expression as to whether the toxin is actually a poison or a substance foreign to the central nervous system or whether it is an excess or a deficiency of some substance normally metabolized by the liver.

The view that the "toxins" are elaborated by the damaged liver itself was upheld by Frerichs (11), Stadie and van Slyke (90), Mason and Davidson (107), Bollman and Mann (74), Heyd (108), Snell and Butts (99), Amatuzio and Nesbitt (98), and Walshe (61). Since the liver has many functions it is not surprising that many substances have been considered at fault. Errors in the metabolism of carbohydrates, amino acids and copper have been hypothecated. Frerichs in 1860 believed hypoglycaemia was the cause of the cerebral coma. Mann in 1927 showed that hypoglycaemia does occur following hepatectomy and that the administration of glucose relieves the condition. Snell and Butt (100) noted an increase in lactic and pyruvic acid and postulated a defect in the aerobic metabolism of carbohydrate. Stadie and van Slyke (90) believed the liver underwent autolysis and was converted into amino acids and peptides. Schiller (109) believed the liver unable to cope with amino acids when damaged. Cumings (58) observed a disturbance in the metabolism of copper in Wilson's disease and postulated an abnormality of copper metabolism as the underlying factor. Walshe (61) considered the underlying defect as an error in the metabolism of glutamic acid.

To account for the genetic aspects of Wilson's disease, Hall (34), in 1921, Bielschowsky and Hallervorden (110), in 1931, felt that the cerebral and liver changes were both expressions of a heredodegenerative abiotrophy. The presence of the giant glial cells of Alzheimer was regarded as a blastomatous process secondary to genetically determined degenerative factors. Rossle (111), in 1930, regarded hepatolenticular degeneration as a constitutional anomaly of metabolism but did not elaborate on the metabolite he felt was involved.

Many important discoveries made in recent years have perhaps been deprived of their rightful place in a historical account. At this stage of our knowledge, however, it is difficult to assess that which is important from the historical standpoint and it is perhaps better to discuss such matters under appropriate headings. With this background the reader can appreciate the provocative and intriguing nature of this relationship. Although in the chapters to follow some of the men who made this history will be mentioned again, emphasis will be on those individuals of recent years who have contributed so heavily to this relationship.

Chapter II

THE LIVER

INTRODUCTION

Much has been written in recent years on the matter of liver-brain relationships by the internist and surgeon but little by the neurologist. The last great contribution by one of neurological interests was that of Kinnier Wilson in 1912 (26, 27). The reason for this would seem to be due to the fact that individuals in such a predicament develop hepatic symptoms first and are cared for by the internists and practitioners on various medical services throughout the country. This, however, has in no way lessened the interest of either specialist. It is quite obvious that neither the internist nor the neurologist will solve the problem alone since the ultimate answer lies in the depths of biochemical phenomena and the internist has not the time to delve into the complexities of brain metabolism nor has the neurologist the time to delve into the fine details of hepatic metabolism. An alliance and cooperative research between the internist, surgeon, neurologist and bio-chemist is the only answer to a successful solution of this relation-ship.

The case material upon which the clinical aspect of this relation-ship is based was culled from the medical and neurological serv-ices of the University of Minnesota Hospitals and so in part this study is a cooperative one. The material consists basically of 40 patients with hepatic disease who did not progress to or develop coma and 42 patients who did have coma and expired in that state. This last group also constitutes the material for the neuro-pathologic studies as discussed in Chapter VII.

THE PROBLEM

Some of the historical background of this relationship has been discussed including the proposed theories. Although there is much evidence and support for the contention that the cerebral symptoms develop as result of a failing liver, there is a belief that this is not the sole cause in all cases of a faulty relationship between these two organs. The secondary cerebral involvement is probably true in most instances of hepatic coma but does not necessarily apply to Wilson's disease. The postulates are then, that the liver is the initial seat of disease and that the nervous system is involved secondarily. An exception to this relationship is to be found in Wilson's disease in which both organs are involved by a common denominator, not simultaneously but independently. In either case one must seek some answers in the liver and endeavour to determine the factors peculiar to the liver which result in defects in brain function.

THE LIVER: A BRIEF REVIEW

In a monograph such as this, only a brief review of the liver, its anatomy, its functions and pathology, is possible and even necessary. Details which the reader may desire to know can be found in any of the excellent texts on liver disease such as that of Schiff (112), Lichtman (113) and Sherlock (114) to mention but three of the more recent ones. The following brief account of the liver is given as a necessary background to an understanding of this relationship and also for the neurologist and others whose knowledge of the liver may be wanting.

Functions

The liver, interposed between the gastrointestinal system and the cardiovascular system, like a gaint sieve, has as a consequence many functions. In general the organ functions in the conversion of ingested food substances to utilizable metabolic substances, the excretion of certain catabolic substances, the maintenance of a balance between anabolism and catabolism and the "detoxification" of "toxins." It is not correct to either anatomically isolate the liver in assessing its functions any more than one can isolate the brain and determine its functions. The liver should be considered in conjunction with the spleen, pancreas, intestine and kidney for without these organs it would not function at all. Many functions have been attributed to the liver. Knisely (115) utilizing

TABLE I

Functions of the Liver

1. The formation and excretion of bile acids.
2. The formation and excretion of bilirubin.
3. The metabolism of nutrient substances.
4. The conversion of glucose to glycogen and the reconversion of glycogen to glucose.
5. The storage of glycogen.
6. The synthesis of urea.
7. The formation and maintenance of serum proteins.
8. The metabolism of lipoproteins.
9. The metabolism and esterification of cholesterol.
10. The metalization of proteins.
11. The amination, deamination, transamination of proteins, amino acids and peptides.
12. The metabolism of hormones.
13. The metabolism of phosphatases, oxidases, dehydrogenases and other enzymes.
14. The degradation and resynthesis of hemoglobin.
15. The metabolism of prothrombin, thrombin and other blood coagulation factors.
16. The metabolism of copper-albumin fractions.
17. The metabolism of ceruloplasmin.
18. The metabolism of iron.
19. The metabolism of zinc.
20. The neutralization of foreign metals.
21. The formation of lymph.
22. The metabolism of porphyrins.
23. The detoxication and inactivation of metabolic waste and foreign materials.
24. Reservoir of blood.
25. Water and electrocyte metabolism.
26. The metabolism of ammonia.
27. The metabolism of mucoproteins.
28. The formation of antibodies.
29. The metabolism of vitamins A, B, C, D, E, K.

a library survey undertaken by a biochemist mentioned that there were 500 clinical reactions believed to occur in the liver. While such a prodigious number may be correct one would have to consider even the transfer of one hydrogen or oxygen atom from one compound to another as a separate reaction. It is unlikely that one could categorize these reactions in a practical clinical list. Every one agrees, however, that the liver has multiple functions. Table I is a generalized and abbreviated list of hepatic functions.

Anatomy

Its anatomical configuration is well known to all. Emphasis should be placed upon the dual blood supply via the hepatic artery and the portal vein system. The latter is of special import since it conveys to the liver, blood from the spleen, stomach, pancreas, duodenum, the small intestine, colon and gallbladder. This venous collecting system is important not only because there is a mixing of this blood with arterial blood in the liver but also because in hepatic disease its flow may become defective promoting thereby

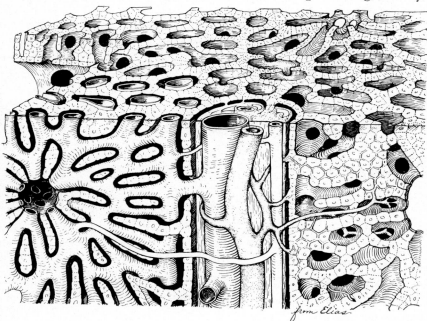

Fig. 8. Modern concept of the liver microscopic anatomy. A portal tract is apparent in the foreground. Glissonii's liver (Fig. 6) shows his appreciation of the venous system within the liver but the lack of the microscope denied him the knowledge of the allular anatomy of the liver.

the development of collateral channels via the umbilical, esophageal and diaphragmatic venous systems. Venous connections between esophagus, diaphragm, abdominal wall, omentum and liver although not normally important or used, become so in the face of hepatic failure. The vein itself is valveless and is formed by the union of the splenic and superior mesenteric veins. Sudden occlusion of this vein is not necessarily fatal but this would depend upon the speed of development of collateral channels. The pressure in the portal vein is normally low but may be raised during portal vein constriction, portal vein anastomosis, and cirrhosis. The egress of blood from the liver is via the hepatic veins to the inferior vena cava.

The microscopic aspects of the liver have been the object of intensive study and now is under the scrutiny of the electron microscope and other devices which may change the current concepts somewhat. Its current anatomy is depicted in Figure 8. This in passing may be compared with the early cut from Glissonii as shown in Figure 6. The cut surface of the liver shows the lobular unit with a central vein, the radiating cords of liver cells and the peripherally located portal tract consisting of hepatic arterial twigs, portal venous twigs and bile duct collecting units (Fig. 8). Some connective tissue in the periphery of the lobule completes the basic unit of which the liver is composed. The organ is kept united by the capsule of Glisson.

Function Tests

The search for tests which would both foretell early hepatic disease and tests which would correlate with the severity or degree of hepatic disease have been the object of liver investigators and clinicians for more than a hundred years. Obviously because of its multifunctioning capacity one test could not be expected to accomplish this end. As a consequence many tests have been devised and designed to measure a certain function of the liver. Liver function tests have been grouped into batteries in an attempt to differentiate the types of hepatic disease. In general there are three categories of liver function tests, e.g., tests of excretory capacity, tests of ability to synthesize compounds, and a miscellaneous test group of special functions. Listed here are some of the more reliable and frequently used tests of liver function. The details of the test procedure can be found in appropriate texts. The effects of some of these compounds upon the nervous system is found in the last chapter.

Test of Bile Pigment Metabolism: *Van den Bergh Reaction.* This is a routine procedure in the investigation of jaundice and provides some confirmation of a clinical impression. This test is more informative diagnostically and prognostically when repeated serially. An increase in serum bilirubin has always been associated with liver disease. The source of the bilirubin is hemoglobin and many organs of the body contribute to its formation. That the liver is not the sole producer of bilirubin is demonstrated in hepatectomized dogs which still manufacture bilirubin. The Kupffer cells of the liver, the bone marrow and the spleen also contribute to the serum pool. Mann feels the bone marrow is the most important site. Bilirubin can be produced acellularly and Leschke (116) has produced this substance by addition of cell free cerebrospinal fluid to the red blood cells. This, however, is not a normal method of production. The main function of the liver lies in the excretion of bilirubin which is carried out by the polygonal parenchymal cells. Any type of hepatic disease is associated with elevations of the serum bilirubin. Two forms of the test are known; the direct, a measure of the bilirubin which has regurgitated from the biliary tree and the indirect, a measure of the bilirubin retained in blood stream and which has not passed through the liver cells. In obstructive jaundice the van den Bergh reaction is direct and strongly positive while in hemolytic jaundice the bilirubin is formed more rapidly than it can be excreted by the liver and the van den Bergh reagent gives an indirect reaction. Himsworth (117) is of the opinion that there is no good laboratory means of differentiating extra-hepatic obstruction from inflammatory jaundice. The values are expressed in milligrams per cent with the normal 1 minute direct being 0.2 and the total serum bilirubin being 0.8-1.0 milligrams per 100 cubic centimeters of blood. As seen in the last chapter, bilirubin may play some role in the production of nervous system symptoms.

Urobilinogen. Bilirubin excreted into the bile is converted by the intestinal flora into urobilinogen which substance is partly reabsorbed, reaches the liver and is eventually excreted into the urine. Two forms of urobilinogens are present in both urine and feces, namely sterco and mesobilirubinogen. Elevation of the urinary uribilinogen occurs in any type of hepatocellular damage according to Watson and Hoffbauer (118). It is elevated in cirrhosis of both types and fatty metamorphosis of the liver according to Popper *et al.* (119). The values are expressed either in

Ehrlich units or milligrams per 24 hours. The effects of this substance on brain function have not been evaluated.

Coproporphyrin: Hoffbauer (120) has shown that the coproporphyrin excretion is a very sensitive index of liver dysfunction. The urinary coproporphyrin excretion is elevated in cirrhosis according to Watson, Sutherland and Hawkinson (121) and in hepatitis, Watson, Hawkinson, and Capps (122). The upper limit of urinary coproporphyrin excretion is 250 to 300 gamma per 24 hours. The porphyrins are important to brain metabolism.

Serum Proteins: The liver is the site of formation of the plasma proteins notably prothrombin, fibrinogen, and albumin. The source of the serum globulins has provoked considerable disagreement. Most authorities now agree on the liver as the site of serum albumin and most of the serum globulins. Popper, Huerga, Steigmann and Sladki (123) believe the globulins are formed by the reticuloendothelial, plasma and Kupfer cells. An elevation of the gamma globulin represents stimulation of the Kupfer cells. Spellberg, Cohn, Wolfson and Shore (124) did serum albumin, alpha, beta and gamma globulin determinations (in addition to other liver function studies) in 28 patients of varied liver pathology and found an elevation of the gamma globulin as the most frequently encountered abnormality. They concluded that the serum globulins are a better index of liver dysfunction than the flocculation tests which depend upon an altered gamma globulin. Support of this is also found in studies by Marrack and Hoch (125) who believe the characteristic change in liver disease is the increase in blood gamma globulin levels. The albumin is sometimes reduced and in severe liver damage the albumin-globulin ratio is reversed. The values are expressed in grams per cent. The range of the total proteins is 6 to 8 grams per 100 cubic centimeters, for the albumin, 3 to 4, and globulin, 2 to 3 grams per cent. The normal ratio of albumin to globulin is 3 to 2.

Thymol Turbidity: The thymol turbidity test was first described by MacLagen (126) who believed the globulin-thymol-phospholipid precipitate to be dependent upon the gamma globulin fraction. Cohen and Thompsen (127) showed that the test depends upon the reaction with beta globulin. Kunkel and Hoagland stated that the test depends upon the presence of both lipids and abnormal lipid protein complexes migrating in the beta globulin fraction. Whatever the globulin fraction involved, no particular function of the liver is tested and the total serum proteins are above normal in 50 per cent of the cases in which the thymol turbidity is positive. The normal value is less than 4—expressed in units.

Cephalin Flocculation Test: This is likewise a turbidmetric test based on the capacity of an altered globulin constituent of serum to become affixed to colloidal elements (cholesterol and lecithin in ether). The test was first described by Hanger (128) in 1939. Good correlation exists between clinical severity and the degree of flocculation. Watson and Rappoport (129) compared the thymol turbidity and cephalin flocculation and found that although the tests agreed in 89 per cent of the cases, the underlying mechanisms were different. The test is expressed in units of positivity.

Alkaline Phosphatase: The determination of the serum alkaline phosphatase is generally considered as indicating an obstructive lesion of the liver. It is elevated in both obstructive hepatic disease, certain neoplasms and skeletal diseases. Much debate exists as to whether this enzyme is elevated because of retention and inability of the liver to metabolize it properly or whether it reflects regeneration of hepatic parenchymal cells. Values between 4 and 15 units are found in hepatitis and cirrhosis. The values are expressed in either Bodansky or King-Armstrong units depending upon the method used. The upper normal is 15 Bodansky units or 13 King-Armstrong units.

Prothrombin Time: Recent advances have considerably expanded the concept of blood clotting and coagulation. Platelets, thromboplastinogen, thromboplastin, prothrombin, calcium, thrombin, fibrinogen, a "labile" and a "stable" factor are all involved in this process. The prothrombin time as measured by Quick's method depends upon the concentration of prothrombin in the blood and upon the rate of conversion of prothrombin into fibrin. Prothrombin, fibrinogen and the labile and stabile factors are necessary for this conversion. The liver as a producer of prothrombin and fibrinogen can alter this rate when it is injured. In obstructive extrahepatic lesions, the prothrombin time may be greatly reduced as a result of the damaged liver and reduced vitamin K absorption. In hepatitis and non-obstructive cirrhosis, it is also altered.

Cholesterol and Cholesterol Esters: Hepatic cells esterify cholesterol. In the presence of liver injury the serum cholesterol is usually elevated and the esters are lowered. Obstructive hepatic lesions are associated with high serum cholesterol values and a relative increase in cholesterol ester. The latter may fall when parenchymal damage occurs and as the obstructive process progresses. The test is expressed in milligrams per cent with the range of normal being 218 ± 50 milligrams per cent for total cholesterol. More than 60 per cent of the cholesterol should be esterified.

Hemoglobin: Anemia is common in hepatic failure and is of two types; a microcytic normocytic hypochromic form of no prognostic significance, or a macrocytic form which resembles that of pernicious anemia. The method of determination and normal values are well known.

Blood Amino Acid Levels: This is an insensitive quantitative measurement of blood amino acids indicative of either hepatic failure to deaminate the amino acids to urea or of the kidneys inability to excrete them. Approximately 85 per cent of the liver must be damaged before the plasma amino acids become elevated.

Serum Cholinesterase: This is a test of the ability of the liver to synthesize and maintain serum levels of cholinesterase, a non-specific enzyme which catalyzes the hydrolysis of esters of some organic acids. It is not a very reliable test and in general it is elevated in hepato-cellular jaundice.

Special Tests: Exogenous test substances have been used to determine liver damage by testing the ability of the liver to either convert or excrete them. The bromsulphalein (BSP) hippuric acid, and various carbohydrate tolerance tests are examples.

Bromsulphalein Test (BSP). The liver is the main organ of excretion of this dye. Normal persons should retain only 0 to 10 per cent of the standard dose after 30 minutes. The test should be confined to the patient who is not clinically jaundiced since it depends upon the clearance of the dye from the blood stream much in the manner in which bile pigments are cleared. Suspected cirrhosis with jaundice is an indication. Serial testing has greater reliability.

Hippuric Acid Synthesis. This is a test of the liver capacity to detoxify substances by conjugation and excretion. In this case benzoic acid is conjugated with glycine to form hippuric acid which is excreted in the urine. Some conjugation is also performed by the kidneys. It is an unreliable test and fraught with difficulties in interpretation.

Carbohydrate Tolerance Tests. Glucose, galactose and fructose have been used as provocative test of the ability of the liver to handle these substances. Other organs and systems act on carbohydrates and the interpretation of tests is therefore difficult.

Liver Biopsy: This is a helpful procedure, relatively simple to execute but is not free from risk. It was first performed in 1883 (130) but is now in the process of rejuvenation. The mortality rate according to Zamcheck and Sidman is 0.17 per cent (131) while Sherlock (114) believes it to be greater. Failure to obtain an adequate sample is one drawback not to mention the risks of hemorrhage, peritonitis, puncture of viscera, pleurisy and pneumothorax. The chief drawback is the questionable reliability of the small amount of tissue sampled in comparison with the size of the liver and distribution of the pathology.

Portal Venography: The demonstration of the portal system and collateral channels by venography as championed by Sherlock (114) and others has done much to elucidate portal vein function and dynamics. The procedure is also not without risks since it necessitates splenic puncture.

LIVER DISEASE

Pathological Features: General

At this point a word should be said about the classification of liver disease in general. Because of the anatomical nature of the liver and the progression of one type of liver disorder into another, a satisfactory classification is most difficult. Through the use of liver biopsy the concepts of the pathogenesis of hepatic diseases is changing. Popper (119) and coworkers classified liver damage as either hepatic including viral, toxic and purulent forms, or as cirrhotic including portal, obstructive, fatty and post necrotic forms. Such a classification has at least the advantage of simplicity. Himsworth (117) classifies liver disease under the general headings of infiltrations, parenchymatous lesions, hepatitis, biliary lesions, circulatory lesions, focal lesions and new growths. The word cirrhosis is conspicuous by its absence in this classification.

At present most classifications have been based on hepatic pathology, a fact which oftentimes makes it difficult to assess the original etiology of the process. Although excellent and complete accounts of the diseases of the liver are to be found in textbooks a brief review here seems warranted in order to provide as complete a study as possible.

Cirrhosis: The term cirrhosis initiated by Rene Theophile Laennec is derived from the Greek word *kirrhos* meaning orange. Its true meaning has become considerably distorted and today it embraces fibrosis, sclerosis and has even been applied to other organs. Aside from the finer details of its definition it signifies today an increased resistance. There are many differences of opinion as to the exact pathogenesis of this condition. Cirrhosis is a very slowly progressive degenerative and reparative process involving the entire organ and characterized by a definite increase of the portal connective tissue with or without an increase in the intralobular connective tissue according to McCartney (132). In 1931, Josselin de Jong (133) defined cirrhosis on the basis of three characteristics; proliferation of connective tissue, degeneration and death of hepatic cells, and regeneration of parenchymal tissue. The old concept that the increasing intraportal connective tissue squeezes the hepatic lobules has been discarded. Emphasis has been placed on the regeneration of hepatic cells. Kretz (134), in 1905, was the first to emphasize the regenerative aspect of cirrhosis and that the liver at autopsy is the result of many injurious episodes. In line with this is the experimental work of Mann and Magath (135), Fishback (136), Higgins and Anderson (137), Brues, Drury and Brues (138) who reported on the tremendous regenerative abilities of the liver. Mann and Magath noted complete restoration of the liver following extirpation of 75 per cent of the liver. The same regenerative ability exists in cirrhosis according to Kelty, Baggenstoss and Butt (139).

It is generally agreed that the initial step in the pathogenesis is taken when injury, degeneration and necrosis of the liver cells associated with an inflammatory reaction in the periportal areas occurs. If the injury is mild the regeneration is complete. Cirrhosis is the result, therefore, of many episodes of injury followed by repair and regeneration of cells resulting in nodule formation. As the liver regenerates the sinusoids and reticulum collapse and are condensed towards the periphery of the lobule. This constitutes part of the connective tissue aspect of cirrhosis. As a result of compression and obliteration of the sinusoids, the vascular pattern is so altered that blood from the portal vein may flow directly into the hepatic vein without coming into contact with the hepatic cells producing thereby an internal portacaval shunt (internal, Eck fistula). The blood supply to the regenerating lobule is largely arterial and flows through the sinusoids of the regenerating lobule into the eccentrically placed hepatic and central veins. McIndoe demonstrated a decrease in the actual vascular mass in the cirrhotic liver (140). Kelty (139), by means of models, demonstrated the vascular distortion and obstruction resulting from regenerating and degenerating hepatic cells. This in part accounts for the portal hypertension, splenomegaly and collateral circulation. There is no correlation between the amount of fibrosis, however, and the amount of portal hypertension. The fibrosis in cirrhosis is composed of pre-existing and newly formed connective tissue according to Kelty, Baggenstoss and Butt (139), MacCallum (141), Beaver and Robertson (142).

Experimental hepatic cirrhosis has been produced by a variety of means. Moon (143), in 1934, and Gyorgi (86), in 1944, reviewed the literature and noted the variety of cirrhotogenic substances including drugs, foreign proteins, bacterial products, immune sera, infections, toxins as carbon tetrachloride, phosphorus, chloroform, arsenic, lead, manganese, tar and selenium. More recently diets deficient in choline, amino acids and proteins have resulted in cirrhosis. The macro and microscopic appearance of cirrhosis in humans and experimental animal is almost identical. The cirrhotic state is the chronic form of liver disease regardless of the initiating process.

Most pathological studies of the liver show a predominance of cirrhotic lesions. This series is no exception as cirrhosis was the most frequently observed hepatic lesion. Murphy, Chalmers, Eckhardt and Davidson (144) in a clinical analysis of 40 patients with hepatic coma showed that cirrhosis occurred in 80 per cent of the cases. The remainder of the series was composed of acute yellow atrophy, 5 cases; subacute yellow atrophy, 1 case; fatty degeneration, 1 case, and alcoholic (hepatosis), 1 case.

Although there are many classifications of cirrhosis, the division into portal, obstructive and pigmentary cirrhosis as described by McCartney (132) is used in this study.

Portal Cirrhosis. The gross appearance of this form is characteristic and consists of firm granular elevations or nodules of varying size. The nodular appearance has given rise to the term "hobnail liver" and this appearance also noticeable on the cut surface. The color varies between red-brown and yellow indicating the presence of fat. Microscopic examination shows irregularly shaped lobules separated by broad bands of connective tissue in which a variable number of newly formed bile ducts and lymphocytes appear. The newly formed bile ducts are so numerous and prominent that they may give the appearance of adenomata. The central veins are eccentrically placed and may not be visible at all. Fatty metamorphosis is commonly found. Although chronic alcoholism is the most frequent cause of portal cirrhosis, ulcerative colitis, post-infectious hepatitis also contribute to this form.

Obstructive Cirrhosis. As a result of obstruction, the changes in the liver are progressive. At first there is pigmentation, atrophy and necrosis of liver cells. The endothelial cells contain bile pigments and the bile capillaries are dilated and often contain bile thrombi. Inflammatory cells are constantly present. A gradual increase in the portal connective tissue and regeneration of hepatic cells occurs until finally the microscopic picture is identical with that of portal cirrhosis. Obstructive cirrhosis is much less frequent than portal cirrhosis as evidenced by the studies of Gibson and Robertson (145) who found 21 cases of obstructive biliary cirrhosis in 244 cases of jaundice.

Pigmentary Cirrhosis. Grossly and microscopically this type does not differ from portal cirrhosis except for large accumulations of hemosiderin, and hemofuscin pigments.

Fatty Metamorphosis: The microscopic appearance of this state is quite characteristic. Most authors agree that fatty infiltration is the result of a dietary deficient state and that it is an early stage in the development of cirrhosis. Fatty livers can be produced experimentally with great success by choline deficient diets. Himsworth and Glynn (87) in 1944, Hartroft (88) in 1950, Hartroft and Ridout (146) in 1951, Rich and Hamilton (147), Chaikoff, Conner and Biskind (148), Chaikoff, Eichorn, Conner and Entenman (149), and Gyorgi and Goldblatt (86) have followed the changes in the liver from a fatty degenerative state to one of cirrhosis. The fatty changes may involve few cells or many and coalescence may occur with the development of fatty cysts. If prolonged, the fatty liver is susceptible to further injury. Degenerative changes occur with the development of fatty cysts which ultimately lead to fibrosis. The latter may also result from impaired circulation in sinusoids due to compression by fat cells or collapse of fatty cysts. Regardless of the mechanism, cirrhosis is the eventual result.

Acute Yellow Atrophy: This term in addition to being a misnomer is no longer considered as an entity. The liver is neither atrophied in all cases nor is it yellow. The liver may show this picture in infectious diseases, in pregnancy, following the use of arsenicals, phosphorus, sulphonamides, cinchophen and other substances. A microscopic picture identical with acute yellow atrophy has been produced by dietary means by Himsworth and Glynn (87) in 1944. Since the course varies, a division into acute and subacute stages is justifiable. In the acute cases the patient may rapidly develop intense icterus and expire in coma within a week. In the subacute type the symptoms are less severe and the course more prolonged. Chronic cases may pass into the cirrhotic state. Early in the course of this condition the liver is enlarged but it soon begins to atrophy. The organ is flabby, the capsule wrinkled, and the color varied. Yellow islands indicate fatty liver cells while red areas indicate necrotic liver cells and hemorrhages. Newly formed bile ducts, connective tissue and leucocytes contribute to the microscopic picture. The picture of cirrhosis appears if the patient survives long enough. Bjornêboe (150) regards cirrhosis as being secondary to hepatitis.

Hepatitis: Many epidemics of hepatitis have been reported from time to time. Biopsies of the liver during epidemics show swelling and degeneration of hepatic cells and many also contain granules of bile pigment. The injury is more marked in the central portions of the lobules. In some cases the liver cells disappear leaving only a reticulum. Leucocytic infiltration is moderate. The microscopic appearance may be quite inconspicuous. In fatal cases, however, the liver shows the picture of acute atrophy due to extensive necrosis which is indistinguishable from acute atrophy of any other cause.

Homologous serum jaundice is a disorder very similar to epidemic hepatitis and can develop following the administration of immune sera, anesthesia, and blood transfusions. Contaminated syringes from syphilitic, diabetic and arthritic clinics are frequent sources. While most cases develop following intramuscular, intradermal or parenteral routes of administration the oral route has been the source of some cases according to Runyon, Wright and Beebe (151). The histological changes are identical with those of epidemic hepatitis.

Necrosis (Focal Hepatitis) and Abscess: A wide variety of poisons, chemicals, metabolites of infectious processes and local disturbances of circulation may injure hepatic cells sufficiently so as to produce necrosis. Hepatic necrosis may be either focal, zonal or diffuse. Focal necrosis may occur in a wide variety of severe infections such as typhoid fever, tularemia and poliomyelitis. Such foci are small and do not produce any liver dysfunction. Central or zonal necrosis is the most frequently observed type and is most often due to ischaemia. The central part of the liver lobule being farthest from the aerated blood is most susceptible to anoxia. Some infections and a variety of poisons produce central necrosis. Diffuse necrosis is similar to acute yellow atrophy.

Abscesses of the liver are usually pyogenic, amoebic or actinomycotic. Pyogenic abscesses are more commonly found and may result from the spread of organisms to the liver by way of portal vein, bile ducts, gallbladder, contiguous infected tissues, from other sources as in septicemia and penetrating wounds. These abscesses tend to be multiple, most frequently from appendix and are more often found in the right lobe of the liver. The areas of necrosis may coalesce and form large cavities.

Metastatic Tumors: The liver is one of the most frequent sites to which tumors metastasize. Metastases may vary from single or multiple nodules of small size to massive growths completely destroying the liver.

Amyloid Infiltration: As an accompaniment to chronic suppuration amyloid infiltration occurs in the liver as well as other organs. The liver is enlarged, firm, has a tense capsule and is of a pale color. The amyloid appears as a hyaline material between the lining cells of the sinusoids and the liver cells. Its continued accumulation causes compression, atrophy and disappearance of the liver cells.

Clinical Features

Since the liver is composed of countless anatomical units called lobules, injury to any part of it involves several distinct but contiguous tissues. The symptomatology of a hepatic lesion may thus comprise several components each due to a disturbance of function of a different metabolic system and as the lesion extends the symptomatology increases in complexity and severity.

The general clinical features of liver disease are well known. The best known and most obvious sign of hepatic dysfunction is that of jaundice. While this does not appear in all cases of liver disease it is a feature in most instances. The absence of jaundice in Wilson's disease and in other cirrhotic states even with marked liver damage constitute notable exceptions. Hepatic failure is said by some to occur with the appearance of jaundice. While this indeed does represent failure of the liver to execute its responsibilities toward bile pigment metabolism it does not represent a failure of all liver functions. Since there are great variations in the depth, speed of development and distribution of jaundice it is not possible to correlate its appearance with the severity of the hepatic disturbance except perhaps to say, the deeper the jaundice the greater the liver failure. Body, face and conjunctiva are areas where it is readily observed. Despite the frequency of scleral coloring, yellow vision is a rarity. Pruritis is a common companion to the jaundice. The clay colored or acholic stools and dark urine are other frequent observations that attest to defective bile pigment metabolism.

Hepatomegaly a sign of hepatic disease in many cases does not invariably mean liver disease since body position, diaphragm and rib cage, the points of reference, are variable. The same applies to its opposite state—atrophy. Gross deviations from normal liver boundaries are, of course, pathologic.

Skin hemangiomata, or spider naevi and palmar erythema are indices of liver disease. The former are ubiquitous, fade under pressure only to quickly refill and are composed of conglomerates or varices of new vessel formation and enlargement of existing channels. Hormones have been shown to underly this process. Palmar erythema is sometimes familial but is often observed in liver failure.

The peculiar sweet odor to the breath known as fetor hepatis, is usually an indication of advanced liver disease and is regarded by Watson (152) and Himsworth (117) as a bad prognostic sign.

Ascites, edema of the ankles, hemorrhoids, abdominal venous distension, dilation and increased vein sinuosity and splenomegaly are signs attributable to the failure of protein synthesis, and/or disturbances in portal vein hemodynamics. Thrombosis, constriction, or intrahepatic impedance of blood in the portal vein may account in great measure for some of those symptoms. The failure of the liver to synthesize proteins and electrolyte imbalances due to liver failure also contribute heavily to the pathogenesis of these symptoms. Portal hypertension alone is not responsible but may be a contributing factor. The adequacy of the collateral channels is another factor of importance that is difficult to assess. Palmer and Brick (153) in a study of varices by esophagoscopy found them in heart failure, virus hepatitis, portal cirrhosis but not in association with fatty livers. They concluded that portocaval anastomosis across the esophageal junction may develop quickly is a result of increased portal vein pressure and that varices may already be present in the pre-cirrhotic stage and therefore are not necessarily the cause of observed gastric hemorrhages. The latter is a trouble-some symptom, sudden in onset which quite often turns an erst-while therapeutic success into a fatality. It is a precipitant of coma and usually attributed to esophageal varices.

The presence of neurological signs and symptoms is often omi-nous but as discussed and shown in the next chapter need not be so.

Post-mortem Changes in Liver: The liver like the brain is very susceptible to post-mortem changes which occur very soon after death. Areas of liver in contact with intestines becomes blue-green and the cells show autolysis. Studies of agonal changes in the liver indicate that such changes occur very rapidly and consist of the following; dilatation of the perisinusoidal spaces, dissociation of the liver cords and rapid disappearance of liver glycogen. Hepatic edema occurs as a result of agonal changes in the liver but this is of very little significance.

Chapter III

CASE MATERIAL

T HIS CHAPTER is a connecting link between the preceding hepatic concepts and the following discussion of the clinical aspects of the nervous system in hepatic disease. It is concerned with the liver data which served as the basis for the ensuing chapters.

Mention has been made of the two groups of patients employed in this study. Of these, one consisted of 42 patients that died in hepatic coma and on whom complete microscopic examination of the liver and the brain were made along with detailed laboratory and clinical studies. The other group consisted of 40 patients, none of whom progressed to a state of coma and on whom detailed laboratory and clinical examinations were made. These studies were done prior to 1953 and as a consequence statistical data is lacking in some tests such as portovenography and blood amino acid levels. Since these procedures are largely confined to well-instrumentalized institutions the lack of statistical data does not detract from the importance of the other data to the general practitioner or internist in smaller institutions. The bulk of the patients in the group without coma are still living although it might be expected that they would have passed into coma and expired as a result of further hepatic injury. Despite the validity or artificiality of this group of patients a point can be made—to wit, the nervous system can be involved in liver disease of mild to moderate degree of dysfunction as well as in states of severe hepatic insufficiency.

GROUP I: CASES WITH HEPATIC COMA

The clinical data of this group is tabulated in Table II. The figures in column two refer to individual cases. Of the cases of portal cirrhosis, 9 were alcoholic in view of a history of alcoholic intake. In four cases no etiology was determinable but

TABLE II

BREAKDOWN OF CASE MATERIAL IN GROUP OF PATIENTS WITH COMA

Diagnosis of Liver Pathology	Case Ref. No.		Total No.	Percentage
Portal cirrhosis			16	38.0
Alcoholic	9, 13, 18, 19, 20, 22, 24, 33, 40	9		
Post hepatitis	30	1		
Ulcerative colitis	23	1		
Hemochromatosis	32	1		
Unknown	7, 10, 15, 28	4		
Obstructive cirrhosis			9	21.5
Common duct stones	29, 34	2		
Carcinomas	1, 4, 11, 14, 17, 35	6		
Congenital duct atresia	2	1		
Fatty metamorphosis			1	2.5
Ulcerative colitis	42	1		
Acute yellow atrophy			4	9.5
Hepatitis	12, 16	2		
Unknown	36, 37	2		
Subacute yellow atrophy	3, 5, 6, 38		4	9.5
Hepatitis			3	7.0
Infectious	21, 31	2		
Serum	8	1		
Hepatic abscess	25		1	2.5
Necrosis	27		1	2.5
Amyloid degeneration	41		1	2.5
Metastatic tumors	26, 39		2	4.5

some may have been alcoholic in origin. The remaining three were secondary to a variety of conditions including post infectious hepatitis and ulcerative colitis. Of 71 cases of cirrhosis analyzed by Fagin and Thompson (154), in 1944, 79 per cent were alcoholic and the remainder due to syphilis, heart disease and pre-existing hepatic disease. One case of hemochromatosis is included in this series. Obstructive cirrhosis was present in ten cases in this study. Stones in the common hepatic duct were found in 2 cases, and carcinoma of the head of the pancreas and the ampulla of Vater in 6 cases. In one case no cause of the obstruction was determined and in the other a congenital atresia of the bile ducts was found.

Fatty degeneration of the liver was present in one case. In this study 4 cases of acute yellow atrophy and four cases of subacute atrophy are present. Two cases of acute yellow atrophy were secondary to hepatitis and the cause was unknown in the remaining two. Three cases of hepatitis of which two were infectious and one due to homologous serum jaundice are included in this study. Bjorneboe (150) studied 1,140 cases of hepatitis in an outbreak in Denmark and showed a predominance of females in fatal cases. All of the fatal cases in his series were over 40 years of age and Bjorneboe stressed the poor prognosis in menopausal or post-menopausal females. In this series 3 cases were labelled as necrosis although the microscopic picture differed little from acute yellow atrophy. One case of liver abscess was observed. The abscess was very large containing 600 cubic centimeters of pus and completely destroyed the right lobe of the liver. A previous cholecystostomy was the source of the infection. Metastasis to the liver occurred in two cases and produced sufficient hepatic damage to result in death to the patient from this cause alone as no metastases were detected in the nervous system. Of the cases with metastases to the liver, one was from the gastrointestinal tract and one from a melanoma of the eye. In the latter case, no metastasis to the brain was found but the metastasis to the liver was so massive that at autopsy the liver weighed over 10,000 grams. One case of amyloidosis is included in this series.

Passing mention should be made of the two cases of ulcerative colitis presented in this series. Cirrhosis of the liver with ulcerative colitis was reported by Logan (155), Comfort *et al.* (156), Cain and Cattan (157). These authors felt nutritional deficiencies, toxaemia, and absorption of intestinal toxins were important in the development of the cirrhosis. Jones, Baggenstoss and Borgen (158) found 14 cases of moderate fatty change and 33 cases with severe fatty liver out of 91 cases of ulcerative colitis. Three cases of cirrhosis were reported.

Age

The relative ages are discussed in more detail in the Chapters VI and VII but ranged from 8½ months to 75 in the group with coma and from 16 to 84 in the group without coma. The average age of the alcoholic group was 53, whereas the average age of the infectious group was 36.3 years. Five children were included in the series of cases with coma whereas there were no children in the other group.

Sex

The cirrhotic group is dominated by males in a ratio of 2 to 1. The infectious hepatic states are also dominated by males in this study although the ratio is less with 7 males to 4 females.

Size and Weight of the Liver

The weight of the liver does not correlate with functioning of the liver except in general terms in which it can be stated that a megalic or atrophic liver is a malfunctioning one. The lack of correlation between autopsy size and that obtained by clinical impression is strikingly shown in an analysis of the weight of the liver. The normal weight range of the adult liver is between 1300

TABLE III

RELATIVE FREQUENCY OF NORMAL, HYPERTROPHIC AND ATROPHIC LIVERS

	Number of Cases	Per Cent of Cases
Normal (between 1300–1900 gm.)	12	33
Hypertrophic (above 1900 gm.)	14	40
Atrophic (less than 1300 gm.)	10	27

and 1900 grams. Table III shows the frequency of hepatomegalic and atrophic livers.

At autopsy 40 per cent were considered enlarged, whereas hepatomegaly was noted during clinical examination in 80 per cent of the cases. Atrophy of the liver was found in 27 per cent at autopsy and in 19 percent at clinical examination.

The weight of the liver in this study varied from 415 to 10,585 grams. The atrophic liver was due to acute yellow atrophy while the hepatomegalic organ was the result of massive metastasis from a malignant melanoma.

Many investigators have their favorite "pet" tests or groups of tests upon which they rely. Regardless of the tests used the purpose is both diagnostic, and prognostic. In the latter instance there is a tendency to visualize in the mind's eye the pathological state of the organ in question. Numerous attempts have been made to correlate liver function studies with the severity of the liver disease as assessed by microscopic study of autopsied and biopsied material. Little is to be gained by pursuing such correlative studies since it is quite obvious that the only accomplishment is a comparison of values of unknown significance. Microscopic studies do not reflect the functional state of the organ nor do the present liver function tests accurately reflect the functional capacity of the liver. Nevertheless some general correlation does exist between the severity of the liver damage and the clinical symptomatology. As a part of the study of liver-brain relationships a correlative analysis of liver function tests and the degree of hepatic damage was made.

In autopsy protocols, one frequently finds the adjectives "mild" and "severe" applied to a description of the relative severity of the disease process. While such descriptive terms convey a certain amount of meaning, no effort is made to define the terms employed and therefore any relationships lose some of their significance. Recognizing the inherent dangers in any classification of this type, a simple system of gradation was devised nevertheless. The gradation of severity is based upon the number and percentage of normal surviving liver cells in a low power field on

TABLE IV

GRADES OF HEPATIC DAMAGE USED IN THIS STUDY

Grade	Description	Normal Appearing Liver Cells
Grade 1	mild	80% or more
Grade 2	moderate	50–70%
Grade 3	severe	40% or less

TABLE V

RELATIVE FREQUENCY OF GRADED HEPATIC DAMAGE

Grade	Number	Per Cent of Cases
Grade 1	12	30
Grade 2	10	25
Grade 3	18	45

microscopic examination. The gradations used are shown in Table IV. In establishing this criteria several low power fields were examined, cell counts made and a comparison with normals established. Cell counts and percentages were not made in every case, but were done initially to establish a baseline. Armed with such a system of gradation, albeit inadequate and subject to the same criticism of any similar gradation system, any correlationships that may exist can have a somewhat more accurate interpretation.

The relative frequencies of the above grades of liver damage can be seen in Table V.

TABLE VI

LIVER FUNCTION STUDIES IN GRADE 1 HEPATIC DAMAGE

Case No.	Diagnosis	Age	TT	CC	S Glob.	Bilirubin 1 min.	Total	Pro-thromb. Time % of Normal
1	Obstructive cirrhosis	55	2	—	—	13.4	22.8	93
4	Obstructive cirrhosis	49	3	2—	2.6	17.1	20.4	73
5	Subacute yellow atrophy	61	4	3—	3.0	17.5	32.5	63
9	Portal cirrhosis	54	9	4—	5.1	7.0	20.0	41
10	Portal cirrhosis	69	9	3—	—	.8	1.5	—
11	Obstructive cirrhosis	65	8	1—	3.5	17.5	27.0	38
13	Portal cirrhosis	56	6	4—	5.0	4.6	11.1	47
16	Acute yellow atrophy	68	14	4—	8.6	8.2	15.6	51
17	Obstructive cirrhosis	74	—	—	2.1	5.6	11.6	—
21	Hepatitis	2½ mos.	1	2—	1.5	2.2	4.6	83
35	Obstructive cirrhosis	59	3	3—	5.1	11.0	25.0	—
39	Metastatic melanoma	49	—	—	3.7	—	25.0	120
			5.9	2.8	4.02	10.4	17.7	69

TABLE VII

LIVER FUNCTION STUDIES IN GRADE 2 HEPATIC DAMAGE

Case No.	Diagnosis	Age	TT	CC	S. Glob.	Bilirubin 1 min.	Total	Pro- thromb. Time % of Normal
2	Obstructive cirrhosis	7 mo.	6	2—	—	9.5	18.2	100
3	Subacute yellow atrophy	53	10	4—	5.2	26.7	44.3	53
6	Subacute yellow	46	6	3—	3.2	14.0	28.9	36
14	Obstructive cirrhosis	75	4	2—	3.7	15.8	23.9	85
19	Portal cirrhosis	69	—	3—	5.3	.7	2.2	55
29	Obstructive cirrhosis	57	7	1—	3.0	23.2	33.0	80
30	Hepatitis cirrhosis	56	15	3—	4.4	13.5	17.7	56
34	Obstructive cirrhosis	60	—	1—	4.6	2.6	7.2	92
38	Subacute yellow atrophy	57	—	4—	1.2	4.7	15.0	50
40	Portal cirrhosis	55	6	4—	5.3	2.5	4.5	68
			7.7	2.7	3.9	11.32	19.49	67

The comparison of the liver function tests with the degree of hepatic damage is shown in Tables VI, VII and VIII. The tests which are used include the thymol turbidity of MacLagen, the cephalin flocculation test of Hanger, the serum globulin, serum bilirubin and the prothrombin time. A brief glance at the table shows abnormal values in each grade of hepatic damage.

It is evident from these tables that very little correlation exists between the severity of liver damage and the liver function tests performed. No change is evident in the serum globulin and pro-thrombin time. A slight increase in the values of the thymol turbidity and cephalin flocculation is evident in passing from less to more severe degrees of hepatic damage. No correlation exists with respect to the serum bilirubin. Despite the lack of any cor-relation, however, the tests are all abnormal. The conclusion that it is impossible to correlate liver function with liver pathology at autopsy has been expressed by others. Popper and Schaffner (159), in an excellent analysis of this problem, pointed out the short-comings of current liver function studies. They felt that no test measures a specific basic function of the liver and that most

TABLE VIII

LIVER FUNCTION STUDIES IN GRADE 3 HEPATIC DAMAGE

Case No.	Diagnosis	Age	TT	CC	S. Glob.	Bilirubin 1 min.	Total	Pro-thromb. Time % of Normal
7	Portal cirrhosis	57	4	2—	4.3	1.0	2.1	—
8	Serum hepatitis	57	4.8	3—	3.2	4.6	8.7	19
12	Acute yellow atrophy	55	27.8	3—	6.2	—	—	44
18	Portal cirrhosis) (alcoholic)	43	—	—	—	4—	—	—
20	Portal cirrhosis (alcoholic)	49	—	—	—	.5	1.8	—
22	Portal cirrhosis (alcoholic)	53	5	4—	4.4	1.5	3.7	68
23	Portal cirrhosis (alcoholic)	31	—	4—	—	23.7	45.9	40
24	Portal cirrhosis (alcoholic)	57	—	—	—	—	—	—
25	Abscess	59	7	2—	3.2	15.1	30.4	114
27	Necrosis, unknown	9	4	4—	4.4	11.5	18.7	175
28	Portal cirrhosis	44	—	4—	2.9	11.6	19.4	66
31	Hepatitis	4 mo.	—	—	3.3	4.5	8.1	54
32	Hemochromatosis	62	—	—	2.9		.5	109
33	Portal cirrhosis (alcoholic)	43	4	4—	5.5	7.3	23.9	46
36	Acute yellow atrophy	49	10	3—	5.1	8.6	15.7	—
37	Acute yellow atrophy	5	11	3—	3.5	22.2	34.6	20
42	Fatty metamorphosis	68	14	1—	2.7	1.7	5.3	55
			9.6	3.6	3.9	8.3	15.62	63

hepatic diseases embrace several pathologic processes each influencing hepatic tests in different ways. The authors pointed out that hepatitis, serum jaundice, infectious mononucleosis, dietary deficiency states, endogenous toxins, anozia, eclampsia, and biliary obstruction if prolonged all could produce an acute degeneration of hepatic cells. In addition they observed that this type of hepatic damage, although best correlated with general functional impairment, is reflected in the following tests; elevated cephalin flocculation, thymol turbidity, urinary urobilinogen, and BSP retention; decreased cholesterol/ester ratio, serum albumin, serum cholinesterase, hippuric acid synthesis, prothrombin time and varying degrees of bilirubinemia.

Popper, Waldstein and Szanto (160), in 1950, stated that cirrhosis best correlates with the cephalin flocculation and thymol turbidity. However, the pathological study was done on biopsy material. Popper, Steigmann, Meyer, Kozoll and Franklin (119), could find no correlation between liver pathology and function using 16 different liver function tests. They pointed out that liver function studies were usually done days or weeks before autopsy and that agonal changes added further difficulties to interpretation. Better correlation seems possible with biopsy material. Sherlock (161), in 1946, correlated liver function studies with liver biopsies in 187 cases and noted that the serum bilirubin correlated with the severity of the liver damage. Serum bilirubin levels of 10 milligrams per 100 cubic centimeters or more was associated with more severe liver damage. Popper, Steigmann and Szanto (162), in 1949, using liver biopsy reported that diffuse liver damage correlated with an increase in cephalin flocculation, thymol turbidity, bilirubin and a decrease in the albumin-globulin ratio. No other correlations could be established. Hoffbauer, Evans and Watson (163) compared liver biopsy and liver function tests and reached the conclusion that cirrhosis of similar anatomic extent may exhibit markedly different degrees and types of liver functional impairment. Kinsell, Weiss, Michaels, Shaver and Barton (164) stated that liver biopsy gave only gross information about liver damage and that cellular defects are only manifest by changes in the cephalin flocculation, thymol turbidity and elevated serum bilirubin.

It is readily apparent, therefore, that the estimated severity of liver damage at autopsy cannot be correlated with abnormalities in liver function tests except in general terms. In reference to generalities, it can be said that pathologically the liver in this series of cases shows cellular damage of varying degree and that liver function studies reflect the same thing.

GROUP II: CASES WITHOUT COMA

The over-all frequency of liver disease in this group is shown in Table IX.

TABLE IX

FREQUENCY OF CLINICAL CASE MATERIAL IN PATIENTS WITHOUT COMA

Clinical Diagnosis	Case Reference Number	No. of Group Cases	Total	Per Cent
Portal cirrhosis			13	32.5
Alcoholic	13, 19, 20, 30, 40	5		
Post-necrotic	21, 31			
Ulcerative colitis	16	1		
Hemochromatosis	4, 29	2		
Wilson's disease	25	1		
Unknown	1, 28	2		
Obstructive cirrhosis			7	17.5
Stones	6	1		
Cancer head pancreas	14, 37, 38, 39	4		
Amoebiasis	3	1		
Unknown	36	1		
Fatty degeneration	30	1	1	2.5
Hepatitis			17	42.5
Infectious, acute	2, 15, 4, 23, 34	5		
Chronic	5, 8, 11, 18, 26	5		
Serum	10, 12, 22, 35	4		
Cholangiolitic	17, 9, 24	3		
Abscess	32	1	1	2.5
Brucellosis	33	1	1	2.5

Examination of this table shows that portal cirrhosis was present in 13 cases or 32.5 per cent. Of these, 5 were alcoholics, 2 had postnecrotic cirrhosis, 1 ulcerative colitis, 2 hemochromatosis, 2 of unknown cause and 1 case of Wilson's disease. An obstructive cirrhosis was evident in 17.5 per cent or 7 of the cases. Carcinoma of the head of the pancreas made up the largest number of this group. One case was due to amoebiasis. A fatty liver was present in only 1 case which had also a moderate degree of cirrhosis. Acute yellow atrophy is conspicuous by its absence. Infectious hepatitis, serum hepatitis and cholangitis were grouped under the general term, hepatitis. Of these there were 17 cases comprising 42.5 per cent of the total case load. One case of multiple abscesses and one case of hepatic Brucellosis are included. Some discrepancies are noted with respect to the two groups. Acute yellow atrophy is not included as an entity in this group whereas it is in the other group. Representative cases of this group are included under the term hepatitis. Abandonment of the term acute yellow atrophy is recommended by many clinicians, in which case the percentage of hepatitis in group one would be somewhat higher. It is noteworthy that the diagnosis in the second group of forty patients is made on clinical grounds, biopsy material and exploratory laparotomy, whereas that of group one is based solely on pathological study.

A comparison of the relative frequency and percentage of the

TABLE X

FREQUENCY OF HEPATIC PATHOLOGY IN COMA AND NON-COMA GROUP

Disease	Coma Group		Non-Coma Group	
	No. of Cases	Per Cent Cases	No. of Cases	Per Cent Cases
Portal cirrhosis	16	38.6	13	33.5
Obstructive cirrhosis	9	21.5	7	17.5
Fatty degeneration	1	2.5	1	2.5
Hepatitis	11	26.0	17	42.5
Abscess	1	2.5	1	2.5
Other	4	9.5	1	2.5

case material in this group and that of the group with hepatic coma is given in Table X.

A glance at this table shows that very little difference exists in the relative frequency of portal and obstructive cirrhosis in the two groups. In order to make a comparison, the cases labeled acute yellow atrophy and subacute yellow atrophy were considered under the term hepatitis. Comparing the two groups in this manner shows a greater frequency of hepatitis in the group without coma.

A comparison of the age and sex is shown in Table XI. The group with coma was on the average 5 years older than the corresponding group without coma. It is unlikely therefore that age alone plays much of a factor in the development of, or precipitation into, coma.

TABLE XI
Ratio of Age and Sex to Coma and Non-Coma Groups

	Coma Group		Non-coma Group	
Age	55.7		50	
	Males	*Females*	*Males*	*Females*
Sex	26	16	19	21

Males were in greater numbers in the coma group due primarily to the greater incidence of cirrhosis in males. The reverse, although to a less extent, is true in the non-coma group wherein females are more often subject to hepatitis than are males.

A better idea of the differences between the two groups may be obtained by comparison of the symptomatology and laboratory data. From these points of reference there is very little difference.

Jaundice, hepatomegaly, fetor hepatis, spider naevi, splenomegaly, ascites, edema and hematemesis were present in both groups. Table XII compares the frequency of these symptoms in the two groups.

It is evident that jaundice is present in a high percentage of cases with liver disease and that very little difference exists in the frequency of this symptom between the two groups. A relatively greater percentage of cases of the precoma had some degree of hepatomegaly when first observed. This slight discrepancy may

TABLE XII
Frequency of Hepatic Symptoms in Coma and Non-Coma Groups

	Coma Group		Non-coma Group	
	No. of Cases	Per Cent of Cases	No. of Cases	Per cent
Jaundice	38	90	34	85
Heptomegaly	34	80	36	90
Fetor hepatis	11	26	7	17
Angiomata	14	33	15	37
Splenomegaly	11	26	10	25
Ascites and edema	30	71	12	30
Hematemesis	11	26	4	10

TABLE XIII

FREQUENCY OF ABNORMALITY OF LIVER FUNCTION TESTS
IN GROUP WITHOUT COMA

Test	No. of Tests	No. of Abnormalities	Per Cent of Abnormalities
Thymol turbidity	39	25	64
Cephalin flocculation	32	31	96
Total lipids	24	10	41
Alk. p'tase	25	17	68
Bilirubin l'	39	34	87
Bilirubin T	39	34	87
Zinc turbidity	34	27	79
T. cholesterol	27	6	22
Cholesterol esters	26	11	42
Prothrombin time	30	6	20
Tot. serum proteins	33	12	36
Serum albumin	32	30	93
Serum globulin	32	22	68
Hemoglobin	39	9	23
Urine urobilinogen	18	13	72
Fecal urobilinogen	5	0	0
BSP	27	23	85
CO₂ combining power	14	1	7
Blood urea nitrogen	13	1	7
Blood sugar	10	0	0
Bleeding time	14	1	7
Clotting time	13	10	7

be due to atrophy of the liver as the disease progresses. Fetor hepatis which has been stressed as an index of impending coma was present in the group with coma in 26 per cent and in the group without coma in 17 per cent of the cases. The nature of this factor is obscure but it is felt to be related to some amine compound in the blood. The frequency of angiomata is about equal in the two groups signifying that spider naevi are not necessarily a manifestation of more advanced hepatic disease. Bean (165) relates the development of spider naevi to the inability of injured liver to catabolize steroid hormones. Similar angiomata can be produced following the administration of estrogens. Hematemesis was more frequent in the group with coma a fact which can be explained by the longer course of disease with progressive hepatic

TABLE XIV.

FREQUENCY OF ABNORMALITY AND AVERAGE VALUES OF LIVER FUNCTION
STUDIES IN HEPATIC DISEASE WITH AND WITHOUT COMA

	Coma Group 42 Cases		*Non-coma* Group 40 Cases	
	% Abnormal	Av. Value	% Abnormal	Av. Value
Thymol turbidity	65	7.4	64	8.9
Cephalin flocculation	91	2.8	96	3.0
Bilirubin 1'	97	9.7	87	5.7
T. bilirubin	97	17.3	87	9.5
T. cholesterol	15	172.0	22	208.0
Cholesterol esters	74	38%	42	52%
Prothrombin time (%)	69	68%	20	82%
Tot. serum proteins	42	6.6	36	6.7
Serum albumin	70	2.7	93	2.2
Serum globulin	67	3.8	68	4.5
Hemoglobin	47	11.7	23	12.7
Urinary urobilinogen	42	—	72	—
Alkaline phosphatase	19	15.5	68	26.8

insufficiency and with the development of collateral circulation and portal hypertension.

A marked difference is apparent in the case of ascites and edema which was more than twice as frequent in the coma than non-coma group. While the cause of the ascites is not altogether clear, it is related to more advanced stages of hepatic disease. These signs are generally associated with greater liver damage and less hepatic reserve. The laboratory data in this group is tabulated in Table XIII and compared in Table XIV to similar data from the group with coma.

The most striking differences lie in the average values of the bilirubin, cholesterol esters, alkaline phosphatase and prothrombin time. The average values of the bilirubin the hepatic coma group were nearly double that of the non-coma group. In both instances hyperbilirubinemia was present in a very high percentage of the cases. The lower cholesterol ester value in the group with coma may be explained on the basis of the more advanced hepatic damage, and the inability of the liver to esterify the cholesterol. Seventy-four per cent of the tests for cholesterol esters were abnormal in the coma group compared with 42 per cent in the non-coma group. The alkaline phosphatase was higher on the average in the non-coma group than the group with coma. Again as hepatic parenchymal failure progresses the organ is incapable of metabolizing phosphatase.

While the total serum proteins are within the normal range there is a marked difference in the protein fraction values. The serum albumin is low in both groups while the serum globulin is elevated. The relationship of these values to the thymol turbidity and cephalin flocculation tests has been discussed. No explanation is given for the relatively less abnormal serum albumin and serum globulin values in the group with coma. Both values were abnormal in a high per cent of the cases.

The hemoglobin was lower in the coma than in the non-coma group and a greater percentage of abnormality was found in the former. This may be due to a deficiency of iron or other hematopoietic substances consequent to the hepatic damage.

The prothrombin time expressed in per cent of normal was normal in the non-coma group and abnormal in the coma group. This likewise is a reflection of the impaired ability on the part of the liver to manufacture prothrombin and its precursors.

It is apparent from a consideration of liver function studies that increasing hepatic failure underlies coma. No sharp lines separates the pre-coma stage from coma itself. A gradual transition occurs in most instances. While the liver has many functions and the tests of that function are abnormal to a greater degree during coma than before, it is difficult to ascribe the coma to any one value. The part played by such factors as iron, copper, amino acids, cholinesterase cannot be evaluated in this study because of lack of data. Some consideration, however, will be given these values in Chapter IX.

What conclusions shall one draw from these data? Certainly one can say that there is no single test that heralds either the precise point of hepatic failure or the point of development of hepatic coma. Some such point must exist but its delineation is beyond the capacity of the present group of liver function tests which although useful must be considered somewhat inadequate. In a similar vein it is impossible to assess the functioning capacity of a liver cell by its appearance under the microscope.

Chapter IV

CLINICAL STUDIES: CEREBRAL MANIFESTATIONS OF HEPATIC DISEASE

INTRODUCTION

T HE GENERAL symptomatology of hepatic insufficiency is well known and while the literature is voluminous with isolated case reports there is a lack of detailed studies on the neurological symptomatology. Since hepatolenticular degeneration is relatively uncommon, case material of this disease as a consequence is scant. The symptomatology of this condition, however, is so striking and so well documented that a large series of cases would be of little additional value. Hepatic coma is a more commonly observed cerebral manifestation of hepatic disease and most studies are on this particular phase of the hepato-cerebral relationship. Few studies are available in which cerebral symptomatology has been correlated with liver function and few studies exist in which the cerebral and hepatic status have been compared in cases without coma and after the development of coma. Further understanding of the relationship of the liver and brain is to be gained therefore from a clinical study encompassing these features.

Neurological symptoms in hepatic disease are the result of involvement of several different systems within the brain. Thus, the pyramidal, basal ganglionic and sensory systems are affected. This was appreciated by the early writers (1-3, 8, 9, 12). Such symptoms as delirium, confusion, disorientation, apathy, lethargy and drowsiness have no focal source and are regarded as indices of diffuse involvement or perhaps as defects in the reticular activating, or thalamic projection systems. These premonitory symptoms have been observed by all investigators and there is no specificity for this to occur in hepatic coma since similar findings more or less precede coma of any cause. To Bright (9) we are indebted for an early description of hepatic coma. Pupillary dilatation, spasmodic jerking of the extremities, confusion, dysarthric utterances, forcible flexion of the knees against the abdominal wall were noted. Morgagni (6) was first to record convulsions and Frerichs (11) in 1860 noted convulsions in 33 per cent of his cases of acute yellow atrophy. During the evolutionary years of progressive lenticular degeneration, Gowers (15-17), Ormerod (19), Homen (18), Westphal (13), Strümpell (21) and Anton (25) observed and recorded additional symptoms which Wilson (26) referred to as the syndrome of the corpus striatum. These symptoms, sometimes fluctuating, with nystagmus and intention termor, misled Westphal and Strümpell into a consideration of multiple sclerosis and as a result of this resemblance, they introduced the term pseudosclerosis. On the other hand Gowers and Ormerod disturbed by the emotionality and the evanescent symptoms considered hysteria as a diagnosis. Such diagnoses as multiple sclerosis and hysteria are still made by those not familiar with this condition.

It is evident from this brief historical consideration that the nervous system is diffusely involved in hepatic disease.

Although brain symptoms are the most conspicuous, participation of other parts of the nervous system cannot be denied. Therefore this word should be expanded to a somewhat more inclusive term—encephalomyelopathy. Furthermore the recent introduction of the term—portocaval encephalopathy by Sherlock, Summerskill, White and Phear (166, 167) has served to broaden the concept of this relationship.

Clinicians who have the opportunity to examine and treat patients with liver disease will see some patients with mild neurological manifestations, some with coma and some that exhibit transient or episodic neurological symptoms. The clinical course may pass insidiously and without apparent change in liver function from one state to the other. While some doubts may be engendered as to the validity of classifying the participation of the central nervous system in liver disease, it is quite clear that the symptomatic expression is not the same in all cases and that some elucidation of this relationship may be obtained by an appropriate classification.

Few attempts have been made at a clinical classification of cerebral involvement incident to hepatic disease other than the use of the word hepatic encephalopathy used in an all inclusive manner. Klinkova and Deutschova (168), classified central nervous system involvement in hepatitis into disseminated meningoencephalitis, a polyradicular and a funicular syndrome but did not mention other hepatic conditions. McDermott (169) classified nervous system involvement in hepatic disease into three groups: (1) acute spontaneous encephalopathy resulting from advanced liver disease; (2) acute exogenous encephalopathy in which there is little or no liver disease but with the presence of surgically made porto-caval shunts; (3) Chronic encephalopathy characterized by remissions of confusion, and disorientation.

The classification used in this study is the result of clinical study on the groups of patients already mentioned and on a study of the literature. It is by no means the only way to classify the nervous system participation in hepatic disease, but it seems to reflect that which the clinician sees at the bedside. The individual groups are discussed in the ensuing chapters.

Clinical classifications are always at the mercy of criticism and inadequacy since there is sufficient variation in humans to preclude assembly of all into man-made categories. Objections to this classification might center around groups one and two since a representative of one group may in a very short time be precipitated into the second category. Doubtless, this classification, which is a clinical one, will be superceded by a more reliable one— a bio-chemical one—as developments in the latter appear. It is furthermore apparent that the word hepatic coma is too loosely

TABLE XV

CLINICAL CLASSIFICATION OF NERVOUS SYSTEM PARTICIPATION
IN HEPATIC DISEASES

   I. Hepatoencephalomyelopathy without coma.
  II. Transient or episodic hepatoencephalomyelopathy.
 III. Hepatoencephalomyelopathy with coma and its immediate pre-coma stages.
     a. Secondary to hepatic failure.
     b. Secondary to liver by-pass—Portal-caval encephalomyelopathy.
 IV. Hepato-lenticular degeneration (Wilson's disease).

applied at present and that it should include only instances of coma and not cases where coma does not exist. In addition, there is a feeling for the existence of more than one cause of hepatic coma.

The classification proposed here is shown in Table XV.

GROUP I: HEPATOENCEPHALOMYELOPATHY WITHOUT COMA

Clinical Study of the Nervous System in Hepatic Disease without Coma

The nervous system in hepatic disease shows involvement long before coma develops. Although several studies have been made of the cerebral involvement in epidemics of hepatitis there have been few critiques on the effects of different hepatic disases on the central nervous system short of coma. An evaluation of the nervous system in hepatic disease is, therefore, desirable and necessary, in order to determine to what degree this system is involved in various hepatic states before coma.

Forty patients were studied and served as the basis for this group. The case material was presented in the previous chapter along with a brief discussion of the hepatic symptomatology. Upon admission to the hospital all the cases in this study were personally examined in detail for evidence of involvement of the nervous system. Liver function studies were done immediately upon admission so that no appreciable time lag exists between laboratory data and clinical findings. The neurological examination was done in all patients in the same manner and consisted of an evaluation of the cranial nerves, reflexes, muscle strength, coordination, gait, sensation and mental capacity and visual fields. It is recognized that there are both advantages and disadvantages to this type of evaluation. The advantages being those of uniformity of examination by a trained individual and the disadvantages being those of a prejudiced evaluation. Electroencephalograms were done in six instances. In this group as a whole there was no evidence of any prior existing neurological disturbance. Asymptomatic hypertension was present in one case (Case 35) and hypothyroidism was present in one instance (Case 28). The diagnosis of the liver disturbance was made on the basis of clinical examination, liver biopsy and by exploratory laparotomy which was done in 8 cases.

Neurological Findings in Hepatic Disease without Coma

Neurological examination showed involvement of all parts of the nervous system with the exception of the peripheral nerves. Table XVI shows the relative frequency of the neurological findings.

Examination of this table shows that neurological findings occurred in 67.5 per cent of the cases. There were no detectable neurological signs or symptoms in 32 per cent. Further examination shows the greater frequency of involvement of the pyramidal and extrapyramidal symptoms as manifest by hyperreflexia, toe

TABLE XVI

FREQUENCY OF NEUROLOGICAL FINDINGS IN 40 CASES OF
HEPATIC DISEASE WITHOUT COMA

	Number of Cases	Per Cent of Cases
Cranial nerve involvement	2	5
Reflexes: Increased	19	47.5
Decreased	4	10
Normal	17	42
Clonus	8	20
Positive toe signs	19	47.5
Weakness: Bilateral	9	22
Hemiparesis	6	15
Isolated muscle	2	5
Muscle atrophy	2	5
Rigidity	6	15
Spasticity	4	10
Coordination: Gait ataxic	2	5
Romberg	1	2.5
Gross tremors	7	17.5
Intention tremor	3	7.5
Athetosis	1	2.5
Myoclonic movements	1	2.5
Lethargy	7	7.5
Disorientation	7	7.5
Convulsions	1	2.5
No. cases without findings	13	32.5
No. Cases with findings	27	67.5

signs, and tremors respectively. The cranial nerves as a whole were not involved except in two instances, one of which showed nystagmus and the other a paresis of the third cranial nerve on one side. The reflexes were normal in 17 cases, decreased in 4 and were hyperactive either bilaterally or unilaterally in 19 or 47 per cent of the cases. Dorsiflexion of the toes was evident in 47.5 per cent of the cases. Ankle and knee clonus were present in 20 per cent of the cases. Weakness was more often bilateral than unilateral although a hemiparesis was noted in 15 per cent of the cases while spasticity was in general mild and present in 10 per cent.

Extrapyramidal symptomatology was manifest by rigidity, tremors and athetotic movements and was present in 15, 17.5 and 2.5 per cent of the cases, respectively. Ataxia, intention tremor and a positive Romberg sign were noted in a small number of cases. Lethargy and slight disorientation were present in 7.5 per cent. One case had grand mal seizures without prior history, and one individual showed myoclonic movements.

In order to determine whether neurological findings are more prone to develop in certain hepatic diseases more than others, the symptomatology was examined in portal cirrhosis, obstructive cirrhosis and hepatitis of all types. Table XVII shows the frequency of neurological findings in each of these diseases.

This table shows a greater percentage of neurological findings in portal cirrhosis than in obstructive cirrhosis or hepatitis. The explanation for this is not difficult. The cases of hepatitis were seen in most instances at the first admission to the hospital whereas some of the individuals with portal cirrhosis had had several admissions to the hospital indicating that a greater degree

TABLE XVII

FREQUENCY OF NEUROLOGICAL FINDINGS IN THREE FORMS OF HEPATIC DISEASE

	Total No. of Cases	Neurological Findings	
		No. of Cases	% of Cases
Portal cirrhosis	13	11	83
Obstructive cirrhosis	7	3	42
Hepatitis	17	11	62

TABLE XVIII

FREQUENCY OF NEUROLOGICAL FINDINGS IN ALCOHOLIC
AND NONALCOHOLIC CIRRHOSIS

	Total No. Cases	Neurological Findings	
		Number	Per Cent
Portal cirrhosis	13	11	83
Alcoholic	5	3	60
Nonalcoholic	8	7	80

of hepatic insufficiency had developed. Individuals with obstructive cirrhosis are usually operated on rather promptly and they may either succumb to the operation or obtain some benefits so that neurological involvement does not develop to the same extent.

Five cases of cirrhosis were due to an alcoholic deficiency state. Three of these had evidence of involvement of the nervous system, whereas seven of the non-alcoholic cirrhotics had neurologic findings. This is demonstrated in Table XVIII. This type of case is difficult to evaluate since there are neurological manifestations of alcoholism without apparent hepatic dysfunction. In view of the accepted inadequacy of the current liver function tests to detect minute alterations in hepatic function the entire concept of nervous system involvement in alcoholic states should be reevaluated. It is highly unlikely that the liver is not involved in the various states of alcoholism. In the cases of this group there were no indications of neurological deficit prior to the development of hepatic disease as far as could be ascertained.

Although this represents a small group, neurological symptoms were present in 60 per cent of the cases with alcoholic cirrhosis and in 80 per cent of the nonalcoholic cirrhosis. It can only be said from this that alcoholic cirrhosis does not result in any greater neurological involvement than other forms of cirrhosis.

DISCUSSION

It was stated in the introduction to this section that most series on hepatocerebral relationships have been concerned with hepatic coma. Adams and Foley (60) in 1949 surveyed the nervous system clinically in 55 cases of varied hepatic disease. Seventy per cent of the cases had neurological findings but this included 26 cases of coma. Waggoner and Malamud (48) noted neurological symptoms in 5 cases of diverse hepatic disease and noted the predominance of hyperkinetic extrapyramidal symptomatology which closely resembled that of Wilson's disease. Two of the cases showed alternating mental confusion and a more diffuse involvement of the central nervous system. The authors believed that any type of hepatic disease can produce changes in the central nervous system.

Epidemics of hepatitis have provided a means of evaluating the nervous system in this form of hepatic disease. Cameron (170) in 1943 found 2 cases with neurological findings consisting of paresis of accommodation out of 170 cases of infectious hepatitis. Lescher (68) in 1944 reported headache, delirium, convulsions and coma and felt these findings were due to generalized infection rather than to any specific effect of the hepatic disease on the nervous system. Meningitis was the most frequent finding. Severe neurological signs and symptoms were frequent in cases of hepatitis that ended fatally according to Lucke (62). Lethargy, coma, excitement, restlessness, delirium, scanning speech, weakness and increased reflexes were noted to develop 10 days before death in 83 per cent of the cases reported. Spence and Ogilvie (171) in 1927 found lethargy, stupor, shrieking, crying and convulsions in 16 out of 25 cases of acute yellow atrophy. Dysphagia, nasal speech, palsy of the sixth cranial nerve are also noted in these cases. Muscular rigidity, hyperactive reflexes, dorsiflexion of the toes on plantar stimulation and choreiform movements were reported by Stokes, Owens and Hohnes (63). Dozarets and Belousova (172) reported apathy, stupor, ataxia, hyporeflexia, and paresis in hepatitis and in most instances the changes were reversible.

Leibowitz and Gorman (65) grouped the neurological symptoms of hepatitis into meningeal, encephalitic, polyneuritic and myelitic. The authors found one case of meningitis out of 1365 cases gleaned from the literature. The meningeal signs usually appear before the onset of jaundice. Encephalitis, polyneuritis and myelitis are not common. Byrne and Taylor (67) reported on 5 cases of infectious hepatitis with neurological findings which included parasthesias of the arms and legs, weakness, blurred vision, ataxia, positive Kernig sign, reduced knee and ankle reflexes and an increased protein in the spinal fluid. Similar cases were reported by Houral (173), Zimmerman and Lowry (174), Sepulveda and Peniche (175), Rehm and Brock (176). It is not clear whether such findings in the case of hepatitis are due to the effects of hepatic damage or due to a concomitant viral invasion of the nervous system. The possibility of two coincidental diseases seems remote. Hepatotropism and neurotropism occur in some viral diseases. The virus of yellow fever is an example and the viruses of measles, mumps, chicken pox are known to affect the skin and the nervous system. Weinstein and Davidson (177) reported on neurologic changes in the pre-icteric phase of hepatitis. They noted headache, stiff neck, photophobia, blurred vision, parasthesias, hypoactive reflexes and bladder paralysis. They stated that when such signs appear in the pre-icteric phase the liver is often overlooked. The authors felt that the neurological changes were most marked when there was little evidence of hepatic damage and that the neurological findings disappeared when the hepatic damage was more severe. This relationship between encephalomyeloradiculitis and hepatitis requires more careful study.

Involvement of the spinal cord and peripheral nerves is neither a frequent nor a characteristic feature of cerebrohepatic disease. Polyneuritis, and myelitis have been recorded in viral hepatitis by Hardy and Feemster (66), Byrne and Taylor (67), and Lescher (68). Fasciculations and isolated muscle atrophy have been noted and attest to spinal cord involvement.

Recent studies in hepatitis by Cooper (178) using electrophoresis have shown an increase in alpha, beta, gamma and c-reactive proteins and a decrease in seromucoid proteins in the serum. Schaffner, Scherbel and Lytle (179) have demonstrated a reduction in glycoproteins in hepatitis and hyper-gamma globulinemia has been reported in hepatitis by Martin, and Davies (180). The bilirubin content of the cerebrospinal fluid in jaundiced patients was measured by Berman, Lapham and Pastore (181) and found to be detectable in the spinal fluid in a matter of days even with moderate serum elevations.

Cardon and Atlas (182), in 1943, examined the sera of 4,370 patients and found 54 with hyperproteinemia. Of these, the majority had hepatic disease and hyperglobulinemia was often found. Bing and Neel (183, 184), in 1936 and 1937, reported 3 cases of hyperglobulinemia with changes in the central nervous system. One case had primarily spinal cord symptomatology and was clinically diagnosed as thrombosis of the anterior spinal artery. Another case had positive Babinski reflexes and a left hemiparesis. At autopsy the brain contained gemistocytic astrocytes, Alzheimer cells, glial proliferation and some demyelination. The liver showed fatty degeneration. Although the role of protein metabolism in brain function is obscure it is mentioned at this point to emphasize that newer instrumentation and techniques—mostly biochemical —have added to our knowledge and that perhaps some relationship exists between brain function and protein metabolism.

Hemochromatosis has no particular liver function profile. The abnormal tests are the same as in portal cirrhosis of any type. Diabetes is evident as a rule, but in Case 28 no diabetes could be demonstrated despite other manifestations of the disease. Two cases of hemochromatosis are included in this study. In one case no diabetes could be demonstrated and neurological symptoms were absent whereas in the other case diabetes was present and diffuse neurological symptoms were present. In both instances the liver biopsy confirmed the diagnosis and liver function studies were relatively normal. Hemochromatosis is usually neurologically asymptomatic until liver function is greatly impaired. One case of hepatolenticular degeneration was included in this group of patients. This disease is discussed in Chapter IX.

This chapter has presented evidence derived from a clinical study of 40 patients and a review of the literature that the nervous system shows clinical manifestations in milder degrees of hepatic damage as a result of a variety of etiological agents. It does not seem possible to make any specific correlations between liver function tests and clinical symptomatology or between cerebral manifestations and liver function tests. The hepatic reserve must be of such a nature and degree that coma producing substances are not liberated. The tremendous reserve of the liver is an important factor in this regard. The difference between coma and the alert state is like night and day but no such dramatic difference is apparent in the liver which is accompanied by coma and one that is not.

No explanations are advanced for the biochemical defects that underlie such symptoms. Presumably the defect is reversible and minimal and in all probability the symptoms are the result of alterations in enzyme and ionic systems resulting in either defective synaptic transmission or defective axonal conduction. The answer to this is not forthcoming until more is known about the defects in hepatic function incident to disease of this organ.

Chapter V

CLINICAL STUDIES (Continued)

GROUP II: EPISODIC, TRANSIENT
HEPATOENCEPHALOMYELOPATHY

CEREBRAL symptoms in hepatic disease are often episodic. This peculiar feature was noted and recorded by the ancients and has since been stressed in numerous publications. Substantiation of clinical observations has been provided by the Eck-fistula animals in which this phenomena was observed and related to the ingestion of meat, or other protein substances. Gustad (185), in 1949, emphasized the attacks of transient encephalopathy (hepatargy) which could be provoked by gastrointestinal hemorrhages, urea and certain other substances. This was ascribed to some failure in nitrogen metabolism and the author noted nitrogenous substances in the urine and blood during the attacks but he was unable to identify them. In 1953, McDermott and Adams (186), in a very interesting paper, reported on a case in which episodic stupor occurred following an Eck fistula performed because of carcinoma of the head of the pancreas. The liver in this case was normal. During the fifth postoperative week the patient developed episodes of stupor, confusion, coma, rigidity, reflex grasping, sucking, and extensor plantar reflexes. The onset was always acute, progressed for several days and then subsided as rapidly as it had begun. In a period of 6 months the patient had 16 such episodes. It was noted that the blood ammonia level was elevated 50 to 75 micrograms above the normal. Reproduction of the neurological disturbance and the elevated blood ammonia level was provoked by the ingestion of a high protein diet, ammonium chloride, urea and ammonia liberating cation exchange resins.

There seems little doubt in this case and in the Eck fistula dog that nitrogenous metabolites in by-passing the liver cause disruption of cerebral function. This differs, however, from the state of affairs in the episodic symptoms occurring as a result of liver damage. In the Eck animals and the case cited by McDermott and Adams (186) the liver is normal or at least no obvious damage is apparent although this is open to argument since a liver deprived of its portal blood supply cannot function normally. Furthermore, neither case imitates the state of a diseased liver with collateral circulation since the latter also allows some blood to flow into the liver again whereas the Eck fistula does not. The fistula, therefore, enables the passage of unaltered nitrogenous substances in some concentration past the normal liver into the general circulation. Eventually these reach the liver itself via the hepatic artery although what effect this has is unknown. In the diseased state it is either the episodic liver failure that is responsible for the cerebral episodicity or it is a combination of liver failure plus a by-pass. In some cases it is true that a non-surgical liver by-pass via collateral channels or even an internal Eck fistula within the liver itself may exist without any clinical evidence. Nevertheless some differences exist between the two states. Sherlock *et al.* (166) noted in severe liver damage that the ammonia levels in the hepatic vein exceeded those in the peripheral veins indicating that ammonia had passed through a damaged liver or had been produced by the liver and was, furthermore, in a greater concentration than in the general venous circulation. Conversely in patients with portal systemic collaterals the ammonia levels in the peripheral veins is higher than that in the hepatic veins suggesting that ammonia does not pass through the damaged liver. These facts, difficult to interpret and in need of clarification do not, however, explain the episodicity which so far has been related only to excess nitrogenous substances in the gastrointestinal tract. Although in some cases ammonia seems to be the provocative agent, in the light of recent material discussed in the next chapter, this cannot be accepted as the only cause, since coma or stupor may exist without any elevations in blood ammonia levels.

The recurrent nature, implying reversibility, has been linked to other metabolites. A parallel course between cerebral symptoms and bilirubin levels can be shown to occur over long periods if the case is followed closely. A fall in the serum bilirubin is accom-

panied by clearing of the neurological symptoms whereas a rising
bilirubin is accompanied by progressive cerebral involvement.
This does not mean that the latter is due to the bilirubin alone
since this probably only reflects, as far as is known, the state of
liver function in general. Nesbitt (187) studied the daily urinary
coproporphyrin excretion in 4 patients in acute hepatic insufficiency with episodic neurologic symptoms ranging from mild disorientation to frank psychoses and coma. Prior to and during each
episode of acute insufficiency the excretion of coproporphyrin decreased only to rise again when neurological symptoms disappeared. The authors, however, related this also to the oliguria
that accompanied the episodicity.

Amatuzio and Nesbitt (98) correlated an abrupt rise of pyruvic
acid with coma and a fall in blood levels with improvement, suggesting an inability of the liver to assimilate pyruvic acid, a necessary substance for the Kreb's cycle.

In the series of cases constituting this study there were 7 cases
out of 42 that had transient episodes of coma. Unfortunately no
specific correlations were made with liver function studies for
comparison with the group of progressive fatal coma.

Although this is a clinical classification based on the observed
nervous system symptomatology the inclusion of this state of
transient stupor as a separate category may generate criticism. In
defence of it is the fact that this is a clinical classification and
intermittency is observed in some cases for which there must
be some explanation. Secondly, while correlationships with elevated blood ammonia levels have been noted these are incon-
stant. Furthermore correlations have been made between the intermittency and pyruvic acid levels and coproporphyrin excretion. These correlations do not mean that these substances are the
cause of the intermittent state either but do suggest that ammonia
is not the only factor. These observations tend to differentiate this
from the portocaval encephalopathy discussed in Chapter seven
which appears to have a definite relationship to defects in ammonia metabolism. Before one can determine the explanation for
the reversibility one must know what the precipitating factor or
factors are. We should not err in assuming that the brain passively

follows the state of liver function in all degrees of liver failure. As we shall see the brain takes an active part in this relationship since it is capable of its own metabolism and is not entirely dependent on the liver. This state of transient hepatic encephalomyelopathy is sometimes a stepping stone and intermediate stage to the development of fatal hepatic coma.

Chapter VI

CLINICAL STUDIES (Continued)

GROUP III: HEPATOENCEPHALOMYELOPATHY WITH COMA

THE DEVELOPMENT of a state of unconsciousness during the course of hepatic disease has intrigued men of medicine for centuries. Such a striking and dramatic event was recorded by early medical writers and doubtless observed by countless other individuals. This association has been the subject of innumerable medical reports especially during the nineteenth century. It has also been the subject of considerable speculation and theorizing. We are only but slightly farther ahead towards a solution to this problems now than 100 years ago. Innumerable other problems both in and out of medicine have been solved during this time yet this relationship remains an enigma. Great strides have been made within the past decade but the solution remains obscure.

From the historical standpoint little needs to be added at this time to what has already been mentioned in chapter one since the early history and development of the brain-liver relationship is also one of hepatic coma.

As a prelude to a study of hepatic coma terminology must be defined properly. At present, the term hepatic coma is loosely and incorrectly applied and as a consequence comparisons are less meaningful. McDermott, Wareham and Riddell (188) employed the term hepatic coma "to refer to patients with diseases of the liver or portal circulation who manifest varying degrees of encephalopathy." This would imply the inclusion of all cerebral symptomatology in hepatic disease under the term hepatic coma. Davidson, in discussing hepatic coma in Schiff's text (112) on *Diseases of the Liver*, admits the limitations but uses the term in a similar manner as he says "The term hepatic coma, in spite of the limitations that all patients may not be or even become comatose, is considered as the best and most widely accepted term to embrace all clinical manifestations of the syndrome." It is quite obvious that this is a loose application of the word for it suggests that the underlying defect whatever its nature is the same regardless of the cerebral symptoms elaborated. That many cerebral symptoms occur in hepatic disease short of coma is apparent to any who has studied the relationship. One must not suppose or assume that the pyramidal cells of the neocortex have the same metabolism quantitatively or qualitatively as the thalamic, reticular, amygdalar or hypothalamic nuclei or even that the basal ganglia have the same metabolism as the cortical neurones. Furthermore, neuropathological studies show alterations in the white matter the metabolism of which is vastly different from that of the neurones. In a similar vein the alterations in the glial elements are also present, the metabolism of which is different from that of neurones and white matter. It is this feature that perhaps underlies the entire thesis of this study—namely— the alterations within the brain are diverse and in general implicate three major elements, the neurones in different areas, the conducting fibers and the supporting glial elements, the metabolism of which in each case is different. It is unlikely, therefore, that one substance resulting from liver failure is the cause of all of the cerebral alterations.

Coma is derived from the Greek κῶμα meaning deep sleep (189) and the Latin equivalent is *sopor*. The term was used by Hippocrates to mean also lethargy. The term first appeared in English literature in 1646 being used by Sir Thomas Browne. It is in this vein that coma is used in this study, e.g., a state of profound insensibility, mental sluggishness, torpor and unconsciousness. It does not include states in which coma is non-existent.

In this discussion, hepatic coma resulting from liver failure and coma secondary to liver by-pass will be discussed. No statistical data is offered in support of the latter group since portal venography was not done in any of the cases.

The material upon which this study is based consists of 42 cases of varied liver disease all of which expired in hepatic coma. This case material has been presented in Chapter III and is also the basis for the neuropathologic study described in Chapter IX.

Hepatic Coma due to Liver Failure

The extent of the hepatic lesion or in other words, the hepatic
reserve, is the chief determining factor in the production of coma.
Mild degrees of liver damage are not accompanied by neurological symptoms whereas severe liver disease is always accompanied by neurological changes. In turning to the liver one might
ask what are the significant signs of liver failure? It is apparent
that similar symptoms are present in the diseased but compensated liver as are present in the decompensated liver. The clinician
determines the latter state by the progression of symptoms. There
is no sharp dividing line that is clinically determinable since no
new symptoms appear at the moment decompensation sets in and
indeed coma may occur without decompensation on the part of
the liver although this is the exception rather than the rule. The
degree of hepatic failure in this study has been discussed in
Chapter III. In Table XII the clinical symptoms of hepatic disease with and without coma were compared and attention is in-
vited again to the similarity of the symptoms in liver damage in
the groups with coma and without coma.

Similar generalizations may be made with reference to the laboratory findings in hepatic disease. Again no single test delineates
the point of decompensation and the clinician relies on serial tests
to determine the development of this state.

The lack of significant laboratory findings has been noted by
many investigators (60, 61, 160, 162, 144). Walshe (61) could find
no changes in the proteins although blood amino acids were
elevated. Murphy, Chalmers, Eckhardt and Davidson (144) noted
a rise in the blood urea nitrogen, white cell count, and a decrease
in plasma carbon dioxide. No alterations of significance were
found in the bilirubin, thymol turbidity, cephalin flocculation or
prothrombin concentration. The cerebrospinal fluid was normal
although small amounts of bilirubin appeared in the cerebrospinal
fluid when the serum bilirubin reached values in excess of 13 to
20 milligrams per 100 cubic centimeters.

Neurological Findings: While a detailed neurological examination was made in but 13 of the 42 cases, the clinical manifestations
were characteristic enough so that gross neurological disturbances

such as reflex alterations, tremors, spasticity, convulsions and cranial nerve palsies were noted. It is doubtful whether in the state of coma any more information could be obtained with a detailed examination by a neurological consultation.

The neurological findings are listed in Table XIX. The percentage of neurological findings in this group is 100 per cent as compared to 67.5 per cent in the cases without coma.

Coma was the most frequently observed clinical findings and occurred in 100 per cent of the cases. It was preceded by periods of confusion, disorientation and lethargy in 59, 33 and 19 per

TABLE XIX

THE FREQUENCY OF NEUROLOGICAL FINDINGS IN ADVANCED HEPATIC FAILURE

Neurological Findings	Number of Cases	Per Cent of Cases
Coma	42	100
Confusion	25	59
Disorientation	14	33
Lethargy	8	19
Convulsions	4	9
Tremors	2	4
Rigidity	2	4
Spasticity	5	11
Ataxia	1	2
Nystagmus	1	2
Hyperreflexia	5	11
Clonus	5	11
Positive toe signs	5	11

cent of the cases, respectively. This finding indicates a diffuse involvement of the brain, a feature which is upheld by the pathological picture of the brain. Coma was the most striking and the most frequent feature of hepatic failure mentioned by the early authors. It probably would occur in 100 per cent of the cases if the patient did not succumb to other causes such as massive gastric hemorrhage and indeed this may precipitate coma.

Coma develops through stages of agitation, restlessness, lethargy, confusion and disorientation. It may last for a variable period of time. The average length of time in this series was 5 days with a range of 2 to 10 days. The coma itself in no way differs from coma of any cause. Aside from developing as a result of progressive liver failure it may be precipitated suddenly by complicating factors such as the use of hypnotics and sedatives, gastrointestinal hemorrhage and infections, pulmonary or otherwise. A variety of signs were found on neurological examination. Hyperactive reflexes, positive toe signs (Babinski and other reflexes), spasticity and clonus were found in 12 per cent of the cases. Hemiparesis was noted in 2 cases and evidence of bilateral involvement of the pyramidal tract was observed in 3 cases. The small number of cases with findings referable to the basal ganglia is noteworthy as only 7 cases were observed with tremors and muscular rigidity. This is in contradistinction to the emphasis placed upon the so-called flapping tremor by other authors. There is no doubt that this tremor does occur in some patients but it is by no means a regular feature. The tremor is not present at rest and is therefore a tremor of action or intention. Furthermore, the movements are not simply a tremor but are compounded acts with features of tremor and athetosis. Such symptoms arise from disturbances in the dentate nucleus, the red nucleus and its connections thus implicating the cerebellum in the neurological symptomatology. Tremors are not specific to any disease type or etiologic factor and are better related to location than to pathology. They may occur as a result of muscular weakness and fatigue in addition to the basal ganglia and cerebellar sources. Tremors of this type are seen in a variety of disorders including Wilson's disease multiple sclerosis, cerebral neoplasms and following vascular insults. There is, therefore, no specificity to this tremor. Adams and Foley (190) reported identical tremors in uremia, polycythemia and hypokalemic stupors. It is present in the precoma stages and tends to disappear as coma sets in.

Discussion: The symptoms recorded here and noted by others demonstrate the diffuse nature and multi-system involvement of the brain in hepatic disease. The symptoms, in general, were similar regardless of the type of liver disease and no specific correlations can be made with hepatic symptoms or laboratory findings except that the latter seem to indicate a more severe degree of liver disease when coma develops. This is not always the case, however, as this series is biased in favor of coma and is not a true sampling of the situation as seen by the clinician in all cases of liver disease. This study was undertaken as an evaluation of coma, and the hepatic changes and other factors which precipitate it.

There is no real explanation for the cerebral symptoms in hepatic disease and while many theories have been postulated none have been proven. The theories on this subject as mentioned in the historical account have involved defects in carbohydrate metabolism, unbalanced amino acid metabolism, failure of liver to detoxify toxins, the production of toxins by the damaged liver, accumulation of acetylcholine due to low plasma cholinesterase and ammonia intoxication. The latter has been the subject of considerable investigation and interest and will be mentioned in detail in the chapter on biochemical changes.

In addition to the chemical factors to be discussed later there are other features of this illness that have been mentioned but warrant further discussion. A potentially comatose or pre-comatose individual may be precipitated into coma by sudden gastrointestinal hemorrhage, or by some intercurrent infection, and by the use of drugs. Gastric hemorrhage occurred in 12 instances in this study but in 2 cases this was secondary to gastric ulcers. Gastric hemorrhage in liver disease is usually attributed to the presence of esophageal varices. This, however, is not always the cause of such hemorrhages and it is furthermore not altogether clear why and how hemorrhage occurs from this source. It cannot be due to portal hypertension entirely since the very presence of the varices should act as a safety valve to offset hypertension in the portal system. Furthermore gastric hemorrhage may occur without any esophageal varices. In this series of cases while gastric hemorrhage occurred in 12 instances esophageal varices were demonstrable at autopsy in but one case. It is indeed true, that the living and pathologic state of the esophageal veins is not appreciated at the post-mortem examination because the vessels are collapsed and empty. Sometimes the hemorrhage is submucosal much like that seen in hypothalamic lesions and this may be a possible explanation of hemorrhage in some instances. Regardless of the cause, the development of such a hemorrhage often precipitates coma or causes death in coma. The biochemical factors

that underly this event are chiefly concerned with nitrogen ammonia metabolism and will be discussed in the next chapter.
LePage (191) demonstrated that 75 to 80 per cent of the oxygen
supply to the liver is carried via the portal vein so that hepatic
anoxia might be expected from severe hemorrhage and result in
a depletion of adenosine diphosphate and triphosphate in the
brain.

The use of narcotics, hypnotics and sedatives all of which are
metabolized in part by the liver have a questionable role in the
treatment of hepatic coma. The inability of the damaged liver to
properly metabolize these drugs, allowing their accumulation
often precipitates coma. This possibility is to be considered in
treating the excited agitated pre-coma states.

Infections, irrespective of location likewise predispose to the
development of, or precipitation into, coma. In this series of cases
pulmonary infections were found at autopsy in 14 cases all of
which were terminal and asymptomatic. In most cases the lesion
was a bronchopneumonia and in 4 cases, a purulent bronchitis.
The leucocytosis observed in 15 cases was in part related to the
pulmonary infections. Clinical symptoms and laboratory data in
patients with and without pulmonary infections are recorded in
Table XX. In this study the degree of the hepatic disease was
similar regardless of whether complications were present or not.
There is little doubt, however, that other factors added to the
development of the coma.

Throughout the years there has been a tendency to impute one
substance as the cause of the cerebral symptoms. It is quite obvious that not only are there innumerable proven biochemical
defects arising as a result of the failing liver but there are secondary features arising as a result of the failing liver and there are
secondary precipitating features as those described above. It is no
wonder that we do not know the cause of these cerebral symptoms. Many of these whether abnormally high or low have an
impact on brain metabolism and it is likely that several defects
are at fault rather than one not only because of the polybiochemical defects but also because the brain alterations are polysyste-
matic.

Adams and Foley (60) in a study of 55 patients of liver disease

TABLE XX

Liver Symptoms and Laboratory Data with and without Pulmonary Infections

	Pulmonary Number	Infections Per Cent	No Pulmonary Number	Infections Per Cent
Hepatomegaly	9	60	24	96
Jaundice	13	80	24	96
Ascites and edema	11	70	20	80
Hematemesis	6	40	6	24
Fetor hepatis	5	35	6	24
Angiomata	5	35	8	32
Bilirubin 1′	11	77	24	96
Bilirubin T	11	77	24	96
Total serum proteins	5	35	8	32
Hemoglobin	7	50	14	56
White cell count	9	60	15	60
Thymol turbidity	5	35	13	50
Cephalin flocculation	11	77	22	88

found neurological signs and symptoms in 70 per cent which included 26 cases of hepatic coma. The reflexes were increased in 75 per cent, and tremor developed within 48 hours in all cases that went into coma. In addition he observed sucking and grasping reflexes, muscular spasms, and seizures.

Walshe (61) observed spasticity, muscle spasms, forced grasping, choreiform movements, athetosis, rigidity, muscle fasciculations and meningeal irritation in his cases. Increased knee reflexes, clonus and positive Babinski signs were also observed. He stated that ankle clonus and plantar flexion of the toes is found only in hepatic coma and amyotrophic lateral sclerosis. Walshe also drew attention to the flexion of the legs on the abdomen. Yawning and hiccoughing were observed indicators of impending coma.

Psychiatric symptoms, ranging from the neurotic to the frankly psychotic may be present in the pre-coma stages and be the cause of mistaken diagnosis especially if jaundice is not present or is mild. Disturbances in personality, mood, and intellect have been noted by most investigators. There is no specificity or characteristic features to these symptoms. In this series other than states of confusion and disorientation, there were no psychiatric symptoms.

Electroencephalography: Much has been written on the use of electroencephalography in hepatic diseases. Foley, Watson and Adams (192), in 1952, described the electroencephalographic changes in hepatic coma. The case material consisted of 26 cases with liver disease, 10 of which had no clinical evidence of disturbed cerebral function except for a state of coma. Initially the electroencephalographic activity consisted of short bilaterally synchronous bursts of slow activity in the frontal regions with a spread towards the occipital regions. The alpha rhythm was preserved. The components of the slow activity consisted of a blunt spike and slow wave which were either fused or separate. When separate they "cannot be distinguished from the electrical activity associated with petit mal epilepsy." The source of these electrographic alterations was considered to be metabolic disturbances acting primarily on the thalamocortical projection systems. Bickford and Butt (193), in 1953, discussed the electrographic features of hepatic coma and described 4 to 6 per second activity in the precoma state, triphasic bilaterally synchronous slow activity in the deeper stages resembling eye blink artifacts, and delta (1 to 3 per second) activity diffuse and arrhythmic in the terminal stages.

In 1954, McDermott and Adams (194), described the electroencephalogram during episodic stupor in which bursts of bilaterally synchronous slow waves of (4 to 7 per second) high voltage activity correlated with stupor, random delta waves with deep coma and more alert stages with normal activity. Close examination of the graph presented, however, does not show very good correlation. The heights of the lines of May 12, 16 and September 15 are approximately the same indicating the same degree of electrical abnormality but are associated with exactly opposite neurological states on the dates mentioned. In other words the electroencephalogram was approximately the same when the patient was comatose as when he was more alert. Perhaps a time lag accounts for the discrepancies noted. While this article demonstrated some electrographic changes under the conditions described they must not be recorded as support for the electrographic changes in liver disease because in the case described the anastomosis was made between the inferior mesenteric vein and the inferior vena cava (not a true Eck fistula) and further-more the surgical portocaval anastomosis performed when the liver is normal is a different situation from that of a diseased liver with a collateral circulation. In this particular case, although blood ammonia levels correlated to some extent with the symptoms, they were not considered to be the cause of the episodic stupor because the blood ammonia level was also elevated when the patient was clear and the electroencephalogram normal.

The electrographic changes in hepatic coma are neither specific for this state, nor are they found in all cases. Riddell and Mc-Dermott (195) stated that, "some patients with disturbed con-sciousness do not show the abnormal rhythms attributed to hepatic coma." Schiff (112), Sherlock (169), Whitfield and Arnott (196), deny any specificity for the electroencephalogram in hepatic dis-ease. The electroencephalograph changes in coma are similar re-gardless of the underlying cause. There is always an unfortunate tendency on the part of electroencephalographers to read patho-logical states into their interpretations of the electrical activity of the brain. This is a procedure or practice to be condemned. The electroencephalogram reflects no specific metabolic state but rather an electrical abnormality which may be the result of myriads of metabolic defects hepatic or otherwise. The electro-encephalographer is no better able to state the etiology of coma, or for that matter other electrical abnormalities of the brain, than is the technician who records the sedimentation velocity of the blood able to foretell the cause of an increased sedimentation rate. If used in conjunction with the clinical aspects of the case there may be some merit to the use of this instrument. Furthermore, it is unlikely in this relationship that the electroencephalogram will give any information that the clinician cannot determine by careful clinical examination. Two remaining factors that mitigate against its use are the cost of the procedure and the fact that most interpretations in smaller institutions and hospitals are not done by electroencephalographic "experts."

Electroencephalograms were done in only 2 instances of hepatic coma and in 6 cases without coma. In the cases of coma both records were abnormal but not considered characteristic nor in any way different from other types of coma. Slow rhythms were predominant. Of the 6 electroencephalograms in the non-coma group 4 were abnormal showing slow activity in all leads and 2 were normal. It would seem that little is to be gained by the use of this instrument in its present form in evaluating cerebrohepatic relationships.

Treatment: There is no specific treatment for hepatic coma and therapy is largely one of personal preference. The ancients recorded good results with purgatives. Intravenous glucose was advocated by Snell and Butt (99), glutamic acid was first recommended by Walshe (197), in 1952, cortisone plus antibiotics recommended by Ducci and Katz (198), and Goldbloom and Steigmann (199) also recommended aureomycin therapy in hepatic insufficiency, Latner (200, 201) advocated in infusion of 10 per cent dextrose in saline, 50 milligrams of thiamine hydrochloride, 150 milligrams of cicotinamide, 50 milligrams of riboflavin and 0.5 gram of potassium chloride with the addition of transfusions, 1,000,000 units of penicillin per day and 300 milligrams of alphatocopherol intramuscularly. On this regime, 1 death occurred out of 5 cases and in a later report on 30 cases, the mortality was between 10 and 20 per cent (201). Little is to be gained by a quotation of treatment methods or mortality statistics in this condition for the mortality is universally high regardless of the therapy. Two therapeutic advances of recent years have been the use of low protein diet and the use of antibiotics. The latter have been employed to cut down the intestinal bacterial action and hence the liberation of nitrogenous products into the portal system and also to prevent or to diminish bacterial invasion of, and further damage to, the liver. It may be said here that in some cases this is effective and in others it is not. Their use perhaps would be indicated if one could be certain of the presence of a liver by-pass and of the reproduction of cerebral symptoms by high protein ingestion. In this type of case it might be helpful, but this is not guaranteed.

Studies by Kitamura (202, 203, 204) on the influence of vitamin B complexes on liver function demonstrated that while vitamin B₁ had no effect on the detoxifying function of liver, the riboflavin fraction did improve this capacity of the liver. Riboflavin was also more effective than pyridoxine (B_6). Vitamin B_{12} and folic acid also improved liver function but to a lesser degree than riboflavin.

Najarian and Harper (205, 206) studied the comparative effect of arginine and mono-sodium glutamate on blood ammonia levels and noted that the former was considerably more effective than rise in the blood urea suggesting that the arginine combines with elevated blood ammonia levels resulted in a noticeable fall of blood ammonia within one-half hour. This was accompanied by a rise in the blood urea suggesting that the arginine combines with ammonia and enters the urea cycle. Glutamate was only slightly effective. Doubtless new substances will be tried in the future since specific treatment is not yet at hand.

The general principles of treatment of hepatic coma are as follows: (1) low protein intake; (2) antibiotics (aureomycin, neomycin, terramycin, penicillin); (3) vitamin B complex—intravenously or intramuscularly; (4) correction of water and electrolyte disturbances; (5) adequate carbohydrate and fat intake; (6) avoidance of narcotics, barbiturates; (7) anticoagulants—if thrombosis of portal vein present; (8) care of skin; (9) frequent change in position; (10) catheterization and daily measurement of urinary output and specific gravity; (11) avoidance of gastric tube in comatose patient because of wick effect and depressed cough reflex. Gastrostomy is a better procedure in prolonged coma; (12) tracheotomy-comatose patients have depressed cough reflex and are subject to atelectasis; (13) trial of arginine; (14) enemata.

Chapter VII

CLINICAL STUDIES (Continued)

GROUP III: HEPATOENCEPHALOMYELOPATHY WITH COMA

Hepatoencephalomyelopathy Secondary to Portocaval Shunting (Portal-Systemic Encephalopathy)

T HERE is little doubt that this entity described by Sherlock (166, 167) exists. What is in doubt, is the real explanation for this phenomena. Sherlock has listed the requirements of this condition as follows: a collateral portal-venous circulation, a source of nitrogenous substance (blood from gastrointestinal hemorrhage, ingestion of protein, urea or ammonium chloride, or the bacterial action in the intestine) and a diseased liver. The underlying biochemical alteration has been ascribed to the circumnavigation of the liver through collateral channels by large quantities of ammonia—which (see Fig. 9) cause cerebral changes including stupor, coma and electrographic alterations.

This is a mechanism that could be covered by the "toxic" theory but as suggested in the historical account it is not a toxin in the sense of an exogenous compound that is foreign to the body like arsenic, but rather, it is merely an altered excess of a substance normally metabolized in the body. The mechanism as described appears to be simple and straightforward but its chief drawback is that the cerebral symptoms do not always correlate with the blood ammonia levels. The subject of deranged ammonia metabolism as a cause of cerebral symptoms is currently in vogue and there are just as many investigators for it as there are against it. This fact alone contributes somewhat to its downfall as the prime cause. The theory has been postulated that the ammonia disrupts the Kreb's cycle by combining with alpha ketoglutaric acid to form glutamine thus inhibiting the production of Adenosine-triphosphate (ATP), a necessary substance for brain function. It is

PORTO-CAVAL   ENCEPHALOPATHY

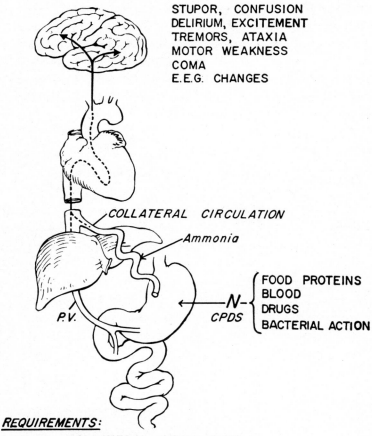

STUPOR, CONFUSION
DELIRIUM, EXCITEMENT
TREMORS, ATAXIA
MOTOR WEAKNESS
COMA
E.E.G. CHANGES

COLLATERAL CIRCULATION

Ammonia

P.V.

N-
CPDS

FOOD PROTEINS
BLOOD
DRUGS
BACTERIAL ACTION

REQUIREMENTS:

1. COLLATERAL CIRCULATION
2. NITROGENOUS SUBSTANCES
3. SOME LIVER FAILURE

FIG. 9. The mechanism and requirements of porto-caval encephalopathy
(from Sherlock).

quite clear that the ammonia levels do not mirror the cerebral symptoms in all cases, for elevated levels are found where neurological symptoms are absent as well as when present. Furthermore, glutamic acid, which is given therapeutically to combine or bind the ammonia, supposedly in excess, does not always relieve the comatose condition. These facts are discussed later.

Before one examines the pros and cons of this relationship a brief historical note is necessary. The early history of this phenomena was born out of the experiments of Hahn, Massen, Nencki and Pawlow (71), in 1893, and Nikolai Eck (207), in 1877, both of whom observed the phenomena of meat intoxication in the Eck fistulized animal. Van Coulaert and Deviller (208), in 1923, Mongiuo and Krause (209), in 1934, and Kirk (210), in 1936, noted similar effects of meat intoxication in the Eck animal. The latter was of the opinion that since the synthesis of urea remains normal in cirrhosis, the ammonia intoxication must develop as a result of the collateral circulation and hepatic by-pass. Since then numerous papers have reported elevated ammonia levels in hepatic coma (166, 169, 188, 195, 197, 211, 212, 213, 214). Walshe (197) first used glutamic acid in the treatment of hepatic coma which not only gave some support to the ammonia theory but which also precipitated some of the discussion and confusion in the literature.

Perhaps one reason for the difference of opinions on the role of ammonia lies within the test itself. The technique of ammonia determination most commonly used is that of Conway (215-217) and is fraught with difficulties for the test must be done rapidly. According to this technique, the normal peripheral blood ammonia levels lie between 44 and 71 μg of ammonia nitrogen for 100 cubic centimeters of blood. In resting patients without liver disease there is no measurable blood ammonia in the peripheral circulation.

The sources of the portal vein ammonia are generally considered to be the result of the breakdown of blood in the gastrointestinal tract by enzymatic action and by the activity of gastrointestinal bacterial and non-bacterial enzymatic systems on ingested protein. Urea and ammonium chloride are exogenous sources of ammonia.

Support for a defect in protein-nitrogen metabolism and excess of ammonia as a cause of the cerebral symptoms arises from the following. (1) The successful reversal of some cases of hepatic coma by treatment with glutamic acid (188, 197, 218, 219). (2) The production of cerebral symptoms in Eck-fistulized animals by a high protein, urea or ammonia chloride intake (71, 73, 75, 220). (3) Cases of episodic stupor with surgical shunts and high protein, urea and ammonium chloride ingestion (186, 221, 222). (4) The precipitation of coma from a precomatose state by ammonia liberating cation exchange resins, ammonia chloride, urea, high protein diet and potassium exchange resins (195, 213, 223, 224, 225). One cannot deny that the changes reported occur and I have observed similar changes both clinically and in the Eck fistula animal. These observations do not necessarily indicate, however, that a faulty ammonia metabolism is the underlying cause even though the blood ammonia level is elevated during hepatic coma.

The failure of the glutamic acid to work in all cases and the lack of correlation between ammonia levels and the central nervous system symptoms (112, 169, 210, 213, 221, 226), catheterization studies of hepatic, portal, peripheral vein ammonia levels (211, 227) have cast some doubt in this theory. In a study by McDermott, Wareham and Riddell (188) 28 patients with hepatic coma were treated with glutamic acid and were divided into 3 categories, *viz.*, (1) a spontaneous group—liver disease without any precipitating factors; (2) an exogenous group—in which the liver disease was compensated but in which the patient could be precipitated into coma by NH_4Cl, urea and high protein intake; (3) a chronic progressing non-remitting course to coma. The treatment was found to be beneficial in groups 2 and 3 but useless in group 1. The authors, however, used the term hepatic coma to refer to patients with "varying degrees of encephalopathy." This points out the difficulties in evaluating reports when terminology varies so widely. Seegmiller and associates (213) could find no correlation between neurological symptoms and plasma glutamine levels and an inconsistent correlation with plasma ammonia levels. Traeger and his co-workers (214) conceded some derangement of ammonia metabolism, but could not correlate the state of consciousness well enough with the blood ammonia values to establish a casual relationship of ammonia to hepatic coma.

Hepatic vein and peripheral vein catheterization studies by White, Phear, Summerskill, Sherlock and Cole (211) showed an elevation of ammonia levels in the portal vein and in all patients studied with hepatic disease and neurological symptoms. However, in the patients with severe liver damage, the ammonia level in the hepatic vein exceeded that of the peripheral veins, indicating that ammonia passed through a damaged liver or was formed in it while patients with a portal systemic collateral circulation, the ammonia level in the peripheral veins was higher than in the hepatic veins. Although these observations do not necessarily mitigate against the ammonia theory, they do indicate that the damaged liver itself has something to do with ammonia and that the phenomenon is not entirely a liver by-pass mechanism. Patients with very severe liver disease do show encephalopathy, but the exciting agents mentioned above do not work and this may be a differential point between the portal encephalopathy and encephalopathy from severe liver damage.

In a study of 3 patients with hepatic coma by Faloon, Anchincloss, Eich and Gilbert (227), catheterization studies of the inferior vena cava, the hepatic vein and the right auricle were made and ammonia determinations along with simultaneous arterial ammonia determinations were performed. It was shown that the peripheral tissues remove ammonia, that the ammonia levels increase as the blood traverses the lungs and that the shunt is of greater significance in the production of elevated blood ammonia levels than is defective hepatic extraction. The increase in arterial ammonia levels over the venous levels suggests that other factors are brought into play—in this case the lungs. The nature of the particular relationship remains obscure yet it points out that the encephalopathy regardless of type is not strictly confined to the liver and that other organs participate in its production to some extent.

The ammonia tolerance in normal individuals and those with liver disease was studied by White, Phear, Summerskill, Sherlock and Cole (211) who demonstrated a rapid rise in the peripheral vein ammonia levels following the ingestion of 3.0 grams of ammonium chloride in normal individuals but a marked rise in those with hepatic disease. Patients with good liver function but with extensive collateral circulation have been shown to have high blood levels of ammonia after NH_4Cl intake while patients with depressed liver function and a collateral circulation also have high peripheral blood ammonia levels. Since there is no difference between the ability of the normal and of the cirrhotic liver to synthesize urea, the end product of ammonia metabolism, this function is not challenged by the cirrhotic liver and is therefore not a cause of the increased blood levels of ammonia. On the other hand the presence of a high hepatic vein ammonia level in cirrhosis indicates faulty usage of ammonia or none at all. The role of the liver in this part of the relationship would seem to be one of three; (a) the liver is by-passed by ammonia-laden blood; (b) the ammonia passes through the liver (reaching the liver either via portal system, collateral system or hepatic artery alone or in combination); (c) the liver in some as yet unknown manner and not involving urea synthesis, produces ammonia. More than one of these may operate at a time. The reduced blood flow through the cirrhotic liver, as suggested by Mann (220) or the relative hypoxia of portal vein blood may contribute to this. Obviously more information is needed on this point. There seems to be general agreement that there is an increase in ammonia levels of the blood in cirrhosis either with or without a portal shunt but especially in the latter condition.

We must now turn our attention to the cerebral aspect of the problem. First of all, the techniques of ammonia determination in the brain are difficult and the values are somewhat questionable. The normal is difficult to determine and may be 0 (zero) since there is an "almost explosive formation of ammonia within a few seconds of death (228)." Brain slices liberate ammonia when immersed in Ringer's solution. The ammonia is a powerful irritant of the central nervous system. Parenteral injections of ammonium salts have a strychnine-like effect and can cause a neuromuscular block. The effects of ammonia on the brain can be neutralized by combination with glutamic acid to form glutamine. Glutamic acid

and its amide are very important in brain metabolism since the
two substances together account for 40 to 80 per cent of the total
amino-carboxyl-N of the brain. Glutamic acid is one of the few
free amino acids of any appreciable concentration in the brain. It
is involved in three enzymatic reactions, e.g., deamination, transamination and amidation which are integrated into one system
whose function is the deionization and removal of intracellular
ammonia.

What, then, is the result of the ammonia excess in this relationship? If, there is an abnormal amount of circulating ammonia in

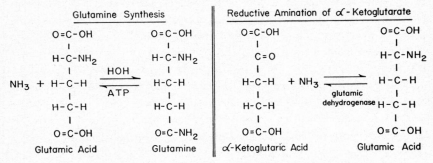

Fig. 10. Showing the formulation of glutamine by the combination of ammonia and glutamic acid. ATP is necessary for this reaction. Excesses of
ammonia may also combine with alpha-keto-glutaric acid to form glutamic
acid thus disrupting the Kreb's cycle.

hepatic disease, and there appears to be, and if this is the cause of
the cerebral changes, what is the mechanism? Is it due to the toxic
effects of the ammonium ion? Is it due to the disruption of the
Kreb's cycle by removal of a-keto-glutarate with a consequent reduction in the amount of adenosine-triphosphate available for
energy reactions? Or is it because of some other mechanism entirely in which the ammonia derangement is merely a companion
to some other biochemical change? We do not have enough information to categorically answer these possibilities. A few facts
and observations are known that shed some light.

Webster (228) reported an increased NH_3 uptake by the brain
after the oral ingestion of protein, urea and NH_4Cl. Bessman and
Bradley (229) and Bessman and Bessman (212) studied the arterial
and venous blood ammonia levels and found that in hepatic

disease the cerebral blood levels were uniformly elevated and proportionate to the arterial concentration. They further noted that muscles take ammonia to a degree parallel to that of the brain. In view of the muscle mass as compared to brain mass this must be a not inconsiderate amount of ammonia uptake by this source. Bessman and Bessman (212) believed that the phenomenon of ammonia intoxication is but part of a syndrome participated in by other substances since an increased ammonia uptake has been demonstrated in experimental shock (230), and in malignancies (231). Since the cerebro-AV ammonia difference as measured by them was zero, this indicated that ammonia was being utilized in some reaction and was not in equilibrium with it. Ammonia is utilized in the synthesis of glutamine (Fig. 10) and in the reductive amination of alpha-keto-glutarate. The synthesis of glutamine, while it would account for the high ammonia uptake by the brain, would also require energy, thus draining off ATP from other energy reactions and therefore producing a cerebral ATP deficit (Fig. 11). If one were dealing solely with glutamine synthesis the uptake of O_2 by the brain would be increased which is not the case according to Wechsler, Crum and Roth (232), and Fazekas and Bessman (233). Bessman and Bessman (234) observed glutamate leaving the brain while ammonia was entering and suggested that the defect in ammonia intoxication is a reversal of the glutamic dehydrogenase reaction with a resultant formation of glutamate by the brain. Ammonia in vitro inhibits tissue respiration and is accompanied by the accumulation of glutamic and aspartic acids according to Potter and Recknagel (235).

The deprivation of alpha-Ketoglutaric acid due to its combination with ammonia to form glutamic acid is supported by the high uptake of ammonia by the brain in hepatic coma and the elevated levels of glutamine in the blood, urine and cerebrospinal fluid as reported by Walshe (61, 197). Against this is the finding of high keto acids in the peripheral blood while the deficiency of keto glutaric acid is on the other side of the blood brain barrier (226).

Not eliminated from contention is the presence of other unidentified toxins from the gastrointestinal tract in amounts proportional to that of ammonia. Oral methionine will precipitate hepatic coma in patients with liver disease without changing the periph-

CITRIC ACID OR TRICARBOXYLIC ACID CYCLE
KREBS CYCLE

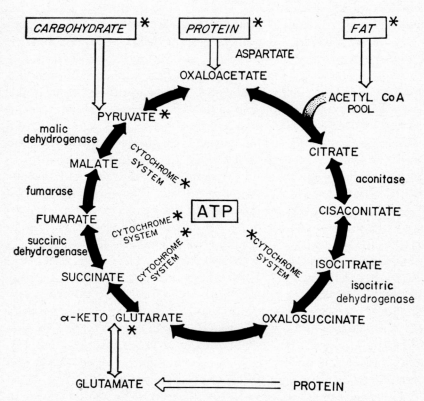

FIG. 11. The citric or tricarboxylic acid cycle (Kreb's cycle) is a series of reversible reactions involving substrates and specific and non-specific enzymes. The cycle occurs in the liver, brain and perhaps other organs. Although all elements of the cycle are important, those marked with an asterisk are particularly so in so far as the brain is concerned. Carbohydrate, protein and fats enter the cycle at certain points. It has been hypothecated that alpha-keto glutarate, by combining with ammonia can be removed from this system with consequent disruption of the cycle and reduction in ATP. This hypothesis although possible is lacking in proof.

eral vein ammonia concentrations (236). Bessman and Bradley (229) believe it incorrect to incriminate one substance like ammonia when (a) the levels are not proportional to the neurological symptoms and (b) the cerebral change in hepatic coma resulting from hepatitis or to a severe cirrhosis vary as does the picture of an individual with a portal-caval anastomosis.

The problem remains unsettled. Whatever the mechanism, there are cerebral symptoms which should be mentioned.

The signs and symptoms of this condition whether or not due to ammonia intoxication are similar to those occurring in coma resulting from liver disease without a shunt. Two aspects of this symptomatology should be mentioned. Quite often this disturbed relationship may present itself as a chronic psychiatric disorder and this has been emphasized by Summerskill, Sherlock and Davidson (237) and Summerskill, Davidson, Sherlock and Steiner (238). The psychiatric symptoms vary from the neurotic to the psychotic and include alterations of personality, mood, intellect and disturbances in visual perception, hallucinosis resembling that observed with LSD and mescaline-like hallucinogenic substances. Depression, cyclothymic states, motor retardation, catatonic episodes, mutism, recurrent manic reactions have all been described in this condition. A second aspect worthy of mention is that the neurologic and psychiatric symptoms are not specific of any particular etiologic factor and in the absence of obvious liver symptoms may lead the clinician down the incorrect pathway unless he is cognizant of them. In a report by Summerskill and associates (237) on 17 patients with chronic liver disease and collateral circulation, 12 patients exhibited psychotic or neurotic reactions. The initial diagnosis based upon the neuropsychiatric symptoms caused clinicians to diagnose such conditions as anxiety state, frontal lobe tumors, narcolepsy, psychomotor epilepsy, multiple sclerosis, ataxia, hysteria, depressive psychosis, arteriosclerosis and Parkinsonism. As a consequence of this, it behooves the psychiatrist and neurologist and internist to bear in mind this disordered relationship as an etiological factor for such symptoms.

Summerskill and associates (237), Hunt and Whittard (239) have emphasized the importance of thrombosis of the portal vein as a cause of the cerebral symptoms. The incidence of such thrombosis in cirrhosis has been reported at 11 per cent. The onset of acute neuropsychiatric symptoms after portal systemic anastomosis may be due to portal vein thrombosis according to the latter. These authors commented upon the "inane civility, politeness and agreeability" as a sign of incipient coma. The abruptness of onset is also noteworthy.

No specific statistics in support of this entity are available from the case material studied in this monograph since two of the requirements were not performed. The cases were studied before transplenal portovenography became popular and blood ammonia levels were done in too few cases to be of any help. Doubtless, there were cases of portal-caval encephalomyelopathy in this group but without clear-cut evidence of portal systemic collateral circulation one could not be absolutely positive. If one takes as evidence of portal collateral circulation, splenomegaly, and gastric hemorrhage then such a diagnosis was present in 18 cases. The liver function studies in these cases although quite abnormal were similar in degree to those without such symptoms. Gastric hemorrhage is not always a result of ruptured esophageal varices as is evident in this series in which in two cases the hemorrhage was due to gastric ulceration. Splenomegaly is perhaps a more reliable sign of portal hypertension than gastro-esophageal varices. In this series splenomegaly and gastric hemorrhage occurred together in only five cases and varices were either not present at autopsy or could not be demonstrated. There was also no x-ray evidence of varices in any of the cases. In all probability varices were present in several cases but without portal venography there is always the element of doubt. Transplenal venography as a procedure must be added to the armamentarium of the clinician as must blood ammonia determinations.

As a brief summary it is possible to state with some belief that there is an entity of hepatic encephalomyelopathy related to defective ammonia metabolism and that the blood levels of ammonia are elevated in such states. Similar forms of encephalomyelopathy may be induced by ammoniogenic substances in high concentrations such as NH_4Cl and urea in individuals without liver disease. Although such observations indeed suggest an a priori relationship there is a need of confirmation for the reason that the blood ammonia levels do not always correlate with the severity of the central nervous system symptoms and glutamic acid is not always a successful remedy. Furthermore as Summerskill, Wolfe, Davidson (226) point out one can expect high ammonia levels in any liver disease in view of the high arterial levels. We must also not assume that this condition is due to a hepatic by-pass and dismiss the liver itself which after all is the reason for the development of the by-pass circulation. That the liver itself has something to do with ammonium metabolism is quite apparent from the hepatic vein catheterization studies. We must therefore find out more about the role of the diseased liver in the metabolism of ammonia. It is quite probable that a combination of liver disease, itself further damaged as a result of the by-pass, plus the by-pass itself is responsible for this condition rather than the latter alone.

A clinical classification has been presented here from the neurological viewpoint and as the cases are seen by the neurologist. This is perhaps less meaningful to the internist or surgeon who view the problem from a different aspect. It is true that the entities categorized may fuse imperceptibly into one another but this is also true of many diseases and does not argue against such a classification. It is also hoped that this broad viewpoint may stimulate more thought since it is apparent that there is a multiplicity of biochemical abnormalities that reach the brain and which may be deleterious alone or in combination. It is safe to say that we do not as yet have an answer to the problem of hepatic coma and that more than one factor is responsible.

It is doubtful that one can clinically distinguish coma due to portal collateral circulation from that due to liver failure alone and therefore there is a need for additional procedures and techniques. Electroencephalography has not shed any light on this problem and it is doubtful if it will. Venography has given us a new pathway and mechanism to ponder over. Further laboratory refinements, and procedures will doubtless give us more information on enzyme alterations and other biochemical and biophysical changes and perhaps even separate these relationships into finer gradations and types.

Chapter VIII

CLINICAL STUDIES (Continued)

GROUP IV: HEPATOLENTICULAR DEGENERATION
(Wilson's Disease)

History

HEPATOLENTICULAR degeneration is the classical example that comes to mind when the subject of liver-brain relationship is mentioned. Although a relationship between these organs was known for many years it was not held in sufficient respect to be mentioned in the neurological texts of the last century. Wilson's paper of 1912 rectified this situation and focused the attention of diverse medical specialists to this relationship. The original title of Progressive Lenticular Degeneration as labelled by Wilson (26) has been supplanted by the term hepatolenticular degeneration and first used by Hall (34) in 1921. The original and unique feature of a combination of cerebral and visceral symptoms has been expanded by numerous case reports and more recently, although the clinical features remain the same, new biochemical features have been added to the definition. The original concept of the disease stressed the symptomatology of basal ganglionic origin and the pathological change underlying this. It is now realized that the disease is by no means confined to this region despite the lenticular cavitation for both symptoms and pathological lesions are found widely disseminated in the central nervous system axis. The hepatic aspect of the problem was regarded as being clinically and functionally asymptomatic but this, too, is no longer true. To the historical background mentioned in chapter one must be added the discovery of copper as a factor in this disease along with the development of paper chromatography. Although recent impetus to the role of copper has been provided by the work of Cumings (54) in 1948, the relationship of copper was first suggested by

Rumpel in 1913 (240) who reported the incidental finding of copper in both the liver and kidney in this disease. He suggested an "auto-intoxication" with copper. Mallory (83), in 1925, was able to produce cirrhosis by the administration of copper and also reported on 10 cases of hemochromatosis 6 of which had a chronic exposure to this element. Gordon and Rabinowitch (241), Cherbuliez and Ausbacher (242), Herkel (243), Oshima and Schonheimer (244) found large quantities of copper in cirrhotic livers. The latter authors noted a three-fold increase in liver copper in 17 cases of hemochromatosis and Dry (245) observed a similar increase but felt this had nothing to do with hemochromatosis. As a remedy copper had been used for 1500 years but it was not until 1928 that Waddel, Steenback, Elvehjem and Hart (246) demonstrated its importance in nutrition. Haurowitz (247), in 1930, and Luthy (32), in 1931, further strengthened the role of copper by demonstrating its presence in the liver and in the brain. Glazebrook (53) reported that although the excretion of copper was impaired in some cases of cirrhosis it was not a constant finding nor was an excess of copper in the cirrhosed livers always present. Glazebrook (52), Cumings (54) and Porter (248) observed hypercupruria in Wilson's disease but Brinton (249) could find no abnormalities of copper in his case of hepatolenticular degeneration. In 1 case of obstructive cirrhosis due to carcinoma of the pancreas Cumings found an excess of copper and iron in the putamen and the globus pallidus. In addition 3 cases of hepatolenticular degeneration showed an increase in the copper and iron content of the same areas. Porter (248) reported on 4 cases of hepatolenticular degeneration with a considerable elevation of urinary copper. As a result of these studies it was quite apparent that copper played a definite role in this symptom complex not only in the development of the cerebral but also of the hepatic lesions. A similar line of investigation on the role of amino acids had its inception in 1914 by Chesney, Marshall and Rowantree (89) who demonstrated an aminoacidemia in hepatic insufficiency. Since the application of paper chromatography to medicine the identification of amino acids was simplified and numerous reports on aminoaciduria in hepatic coma and Wilson's disease appeared (61, 91-95. At present two schools of thought exist as to the underlying mechanism in hepatolenticular disease, one favoring a defect in copper metabolism and the other a defect in amino acid metabolism. A discussion of these follows later.

Clinical Features

The clinical characteristics of Wilson's disease are so striking in most instances that the diagnosis should not be in doubt. Despite this the diagnosis is often missed, due, perhaps to its rarity and the greater frequency of basal ganglionic symptoms in other diseases. It is most often confused with hysteria, multiple sclerosis and paralysis agitans. No difficulty should be experienced if the triad of family history, marked basal ganglionic symptomatology and eye findings are kept in mind. The disease is heredofamilial the genetics of which will be discussed. No better description can be offered than that from Wilson's text edited by Bruce— "With mouth often held open, and a stereotyped smile, or, if not laughing or smiling, a vacant or fatuous look, the patient sits and leans to one side or back, all four limbs agitated by tremor, mostly quick and rather fine; the fingers and hands are contracted in flexion, the trunk is held stiffly and willed movements are slowly performed to the accompaniment of wilder tremulousness. Though saliva may drip from the parted lips, and expressions be almost silly, the eyes are alert and intelligent. Fluidity and fixity of symptoms are both evident to the observer; tremors wax and wane, they leave one part for another, or alter their type in the same segment according to whether it is used or not." Thus the vacuous facial smile and silly attitude is common and quite characteristic. When this is accompanied by tremor, quite often very exaggerated on intention and attention plus rigidity, dysarthria, and sialorrheoa there should be no mistake, for no other condition can mimic this constellation. Tics, clonic or tonic movements, hypertonicity, movements en bloc, muscular wasting, slow labored speech, and seizures have been noted and recorded. Additional confirmation may be obtained from slit-lamp examination of the eyes which will show the classical corneal yellow-green pigmented ring of Kayser-Fleischer and sometimes lenticular cataracts both believed to be due to the precipitation of copper. Occasionally spontaneous fractures occur as part of the hypocupremic state according to Warnock (250).

The hepatic symptomatology is less striking and not diagnostically reliable as an indicator of Wilson's disease. Earlier reports tended to minimize hepatic symptoms and to comment on the paucity of abnormal liver function tests. This is not a true statement as is evident from the reports of Andre (251), Herz and Drew (252), Homburger and Kozol (253), Hornbostel (254), and Franklin and Bauman (255) all of whom found abnormal liver function tests in Wilson's disease. The underlying hepatic lesion is a portal cirrhosis.

Electroencephalographic recordings in Wilson's disease have been described by Stephens (256) in 9 cases of which 5 were normal, 2 of doubtful abnormality and 2 abnormal. Of the latter, one showed 1 per second occipital waves and the other 3 to 6 per second generalized waves.

Ravin (257) recently proposed a rapid and simple colorimetric test for hepatolenticular degeneration. The author believes the diagnosis of Wilson's disease can only be made on tedious and time consuming copper and amino acid determinations. The test is a measure of the serum copper oxidase-ceruloplasmin—a defect of which is a characteristic feature of the disease.

Any doubt that exists in the mind of the clinician up to this point can be dismissed if determinations of urinary copper, excretion, serum ceruloplasmin levels and urinary amino acid excretion can be made. To the original clinical definition of Wilson's disease now must be added the biochemical features as described below. Herein lies a magnificent example of medical progress in which the key to the puzzle of a once fatal disease is at hand. Herein also lies hope for others afflicted with the "hopeless" cerebral degenerations. One has to look on in amazement at the damage wrought by an abnormality of a small and rather insignificant trace element-copper. We must treat with greater respect and study more diligently the role of these metals and metalloenzymes for most assuredly herein lies Pandora's box to this and other liver-brain entanglements.

Pathological Features

The gross pathological features of hepato-lenticular degeneration are well known, consisting chiefly of softening or cavitation of the lentiform nucleus. These alterations are usually bilateral, involve also the globus pallidus and may vary from overt cavitation to a worm-eaten spongy appearance. Similar areas are to be found elsewhere. The caudate nucleus is often shrunken, and sometimes the internal capsule is damaged. On the other hand naked-eye inspection may reveal absolutely no change.

Microscopic alterations are widespread involving glia, white matter and neurones. Of these, the Alzheimer cell is the most outstanding but not absolutely characteristic since it is to be found in a variety of pathological states as previously mentioned. Although the brunt of the neuropathological alterations is absorbed by the corpus striatum the entire brain may be dotted with lesions. Secondary degenerations occur as a result of lenticular lesions. Subcortical lesions in white matter, internal capsule, globus pallidus in addition to the degenerative cortical changes were recently described by Guillain, Bertrand and Godet-Guillain (258). Warnock (250) described one case with severe damage to the frontal lobes in Wilson's disease.

Biochemical Characteristics

The biochemical alterations which have been uncovered in Wilson's disease have now become the most important part and must be added to the definition of the disease. These changes are: (1) increased excretion of copper (hypercupuria) and amino acids (aminoaciduria) in the urine; (2) decreased level of ceruloplasmin; (3) decreased total serum copper (hypocupremia); (4) increased copper content in the tissues of the liver and the brain.

Copper Metabolism in Hepatolenticular Degeneration: Glazebrook (53), in 1945, recorded an elevation in the blood copper and also noted an increase in the copper content of the basal ganglia in one case of Wilson's disease. Mandelbrote, Stanier, Thompson, and Thurston (259), in 1948, noted hypercupuria in hepatolenticular degeneration and Cumings (54), in the same journal, reported in the increased copper content of brain and liver in Wilson's disease. These studies provided the impetus to a study of copper metabolism in this disease. Okinaka *et al.* (260) reported on the presence of copper in the hepatic cells in acute yellow atrophy and cirrhosis but noted a greater concentration in the liver in hepatolenticular degeneration. In addition the authors also found copper in the putamen in Wilson's disease but not in the brains of the non-Wilsonian control cases. There have been numerous case reports on the hypercupuria of this disease and this is now a well established biochemical feature. The urinary excretion of copper in this disease may vary from 450 to 1790 micrograms per day as compared with the normal of 0 to 25 to 30 micrograms per day.

Although Glazebrook recorded hypercupremia in one case of Wilson's disease it is now known that there is a decrease in the total plasma copper. The hypocupremia is characterized further by a marked increase in the direct albumin bound copper fraction and a decrease in the ceruloplasmin or globulin bound copper fraction. This latter is considered by Cartwright, Hodges, Gubler, Mahoney, Daum, Wintrobe, and Bean (261), Markowitz, Gubler, Mahoney, Cartwright, and Wintrobe (262), Mathews (263), Scheinberg and Gitlin (264) and Scheinberg (265) to be the basic defect in hepatolenticular degeneration.

The third copper abnormality in Wilson's disease is that of the high copper content of the tissues an observation which has been known for many years. This triad, of high tissue copper, low blood copper and high urinary copper excretion seems a strange paradox and difficult to reconcile. How can the body maintain high tissue content and still excrete large quantities of copper? No real explanation for this is possible at this time. The decrease in total plasma copper actually consists of an increase in the non-ceruloplasmin copper. This fraction has been shown by Scheinberg, Cook and Murphy, (266), Hagberg, Axtrups and Berfenstam (267), Lahey, Gubler, Cartwright and Wintrobe (268) to have the capacity to pass the placental barrier and it has also been assumed to be able to pass from the vascular compartment into the tissues in other organs. The non-ceruloplasmin copper is therefore able to reach the tissues in greater concentration than in normals. The level of non-ceruloplasmin copper in Wilson's disease is higher than in normal subjects according to Cartwright, Hodges, Gubler, Mahoney, Daum, Wintrobe and Bean (261). The deficiency of ceruloplasmin, then is associated with an increase in the non-ceruloplasmin copper due to an increased absorption of copper from the intestines resulting in copper deposition in the liver and brain. Mathews, Milne and Bell (269) explained the paradox with the belief that the cupruria and copper retention in the tissues may represent different phases of the disease process.

Copper balance studies, although difficult to perform indicate that patients with hepatolenticular degeneration are in a positive balance. Radiocopper studies by Bush, Mahoney, Markowitz, Gubler, Cartwright, and Wintrobe (270) show a decreased fecal excretion of Cu64 and an increase in urinary excretion in hepatolenticular degeneration. These observations suggest an increase in copper absorption from the gastrointestinal tract or a decrease in fecal copper excretion so that the non-cerulo plasmin copper accumulates in the plasma. A third possibility is that of an inherited inability to manufacture ceruloplasmin which affects intestinal absorption or in some way prevents the copper from combining with globulin to make the ceruloplasmin compound and so it accumulates in the albumin or non-ceruloplasmin fraction. The basic defect in this disease with respect to copper, then, is not clear. Whether the ceruloplasmin cannot be made due to congenital factors or whether the liver cannot synthesize globulins with which to carry the copper or whether these proteins are broken down too fast remains obscure. The biliary excretion of copper is normal in hepatolenticular degenerations according to Brown and Porter (271). In so far as the serum proteins are concerned electrophoretic analysis of plasma proteins in Wilson's disease shows a reduced albumin fraction but increased globulin fraction suggesting that the liver is capable of manufacturing globulins.

Cartwright, and associates (261) studied seven patients with Wilson's disease and summarized the biochemical defects in copper as follows:

(1) Total plasma copper—reduced.
(2) Cerebrospinal fluid copper—increased.

(3) Erythrocyte copper—normal.
(4) Urinary copper—increased.
(5) Urinary alpha-amino-nitrogen—increased.
(6) Plasma albumin fraction—decreased.
(7) Plasma globulin fraction—increased.
(8) Ceruloplasmin—decreased.
(9) Non-ceruloplasmin—increased.
(10) Tissue copper—increased.

A more detailed account of copper metabolism is to be found in Chapter X.

Amino Acid Metabolism in Hepatolenticular Degeneration: A defect in amino acid metabolism is also present in hepatolenticular degeneration. A discussion of amino acid metabolism is presented in Chapter X.

In hepatolenticular degeneration, the amino-aciduria (a) is independent of the severity or duration of the liver disease, (b) is not accompanied by elevation of alpha amino acid nitrogen level, (c) shows no specificity to the pattern of amino acid excretion, (d) it occurs in families of patients with hepatolenticular degeneration (Uzman and Hood, 272) and (e) it is independent of the total protein intake. These observations would seem to indicate that the amino acids have little to do with the cause of the disturbance in the liver or the brain and especially the latter, and that the amino-aciduria is a secondary event. As in the case of copper, an explanation is necessary for the paradox of amino-aciduria in the face of a normal serum amino acid level. The suggestion has been made by Cooper, Eckhardt, Faloon and Davidson (94) and Mathews, Milne and Bell (269) that Wilson's disease is due to a defect in renal function and that the cirrhosis developed as a result of a chronic loss in the amino-acids as is seen in the de-Toni-Fanconi syndrome. Attention was focused on the kidney by invoking a low amino-acid threshold theory. This has been exploded by the observation that the intravenous administration of amino-acids in hepatolenticular degeneration produces no change either in plasma levels or in the urinary excretion.

Another explanation for the aminoaciduria is that as a result of copper excesses renal tubular damage occurs. Uzman (273) reported on an increased urinary excretion of dicarboxylic amino-acid peptides in hepatolenticular degeneration in addition to the general amino-aciduria. This observation is also used to explain the aminoaciduria, on the basis of competitive and preferential reabsorption of peptides resulting in an increase in amino acids in the urine in spite of normal plasma levels. Uzman further believes that Wilson's disease is due to a disorder of proteolytic activity resulting in an accumulation of peptides in the tissues. These same peptides form copper complexes causing, thereby, a secondary accumulation of copper in the tissues. The peptides, whether free or as copper complexes, compete with amino acids for reabsorption resulting in both hypercupruria and amino aciduria. He believes the copper in the urine is present as copper peptide complexes. In support of his theory is the observation of elevated citric acids and their peptides, since the de-amination products of these are oxaloacetic acid and alpha ketoglutaric acid both of which participate in the tricarboxylic acid cycle with the formation of citric acid as an intermediate. Additional support is derived from his finding of increased dicarboxylic amino acid excretion in five asymptomatic members of a family with hepatolenticular degeneration. In support of his theory as opposed to the copper theory, Uzman states that the removal of copper with B.A.L. does not alter the aminoaciduria and that the asymptomatic sibs of the family he studied with Wilson's disease did not exhibit cupruria. Brick (274) also considered the copper in hepatolenticular degeneration to be excreted in the form of chelates with dicarboxylic amino acid peptides and was of the opinion that the copper peptide complexes with larger peptide residues in the tissues resulted in the fixation of metals in organs such as the liver and the brain. Additional support for Uzman's hypothesis, that Wilson's disease is a genetic disorder of protein metabolism rather than a genetic deficiency of ceruloplasmin is found in a recent report by Uzman, Iber, Chalmers and Knowlton (275) in which by dialysis equilibrium experiments on liver homogenates in hepatolenticular degeneration the liver exhibited a marked avidity for copper as compared with normals. Electrophoretic patterns on liver extracts from a case of Wilson's disease indicated the presence of an extra function which also possessed high copper binding properties. Uzman further reconciles his theory to the copper over-absorption theory by postulating the presence of a similar copper binding substance in the wall of the gastrointestinal system.

Stein, Bearn and Moore (276) surveyed all the amino acids present in the urine of Wilson's disease. They found the highest levels for threonine, cystine (twenty-fold increase), serine, glycine, asparagine, glutamine, valine, tyrosine, lysine (five- to ten-fold increase). Proline, citrulline, not normally found in urine, appear in large quantities in some cases. Methionine, isoleucine, leucine, arginine and amino-adipic-acid were found in small amounts. There was a diminished excretion of taurine, 1-methyl-histidine and 3-methylhistidine. The authors noted that the amino acid excretion in normals was insensitive to the protein intake, whereas, in hepatolenticular degeneration the amino-acid excretion is quite sensitive to the protein intake and the fasting composition is quite different from the 24 hour value. Their evidence favors the hypothesis that the amino aciduria is the result of a renal lesion. According to Warnock and Neill (277) there is an increase in glycine, serine, alanine, glutamine, tyrosine, cystine, glutamic acid and aspartic acids in Wilson's disease. Emphasis has been placed on glutamic acid and aspartic acids in the hepatolenticular chromatograms by Boudin, Pepin and Calatchi (278) and Uzman and Hood (272) stated that 80 to 90 per cent of total urinary peptide content consisted of peptides of glutamic and aspartic acids.

Bearn and Kunkel (279) regarded the family reported by Uzman as a genetically atypical case of Wilson's disease since they were unable to find amino-aciduria in 35 asymptomatic siblings of patients with hepatolenticular degeneration. Here the matter rests. Two theories have been advanced, each with its adherents but neither explaining all the manifestations of the disorder.

No other biochemical abnormalities are known to exist in this disease. Glycosuria occurs in about one-third of the cases. The levels of iron, cobalt, nickel and zinc are normal in this disease.

Genetic Aspects

Wilson believed the disease bearing his name to be familial but not congenital or inherited. Bearn (280) as a result of a genetic study of 26 cases with this disease demonstrated an autosomal recessive inheritance. He emphasized the frequency of consanguinity in the families studied. This has also been mentioned by Andre and van Bogaert (281), Hall (34), Kehrer (40) and Stadler (282). Bearn and Kunkel (279) in a later report on the genetic aspects of the disease found parental consanguinity in 11 of 16 instances. Seven of the sixteen families studied were of the Jewish race. The authors were unable to find any sign of aminoaciduria in the 35 unaffected siblings of the patient studied. Uzman and Hood (272) found 4 members of a family of 12 that had persistent aminoaciduria, and abnormal amounts of peptides with carboxylic amino acid residues.

Discussion

It is quite apparent that opposing opinions exist concerning the nature of the defect in Wilson's disease. On the one hand, a gentically determined deficiency of ceruloplasmin or an abnormal absorption of copper from the intestine is considered the cause while on the other side a genetically determined defect in proteolytic activity is proposed. Neither theory necessarily explains the relation of the liver and brain in this disease. Is the copper precipitated in both organs independently or is there some primary hepatic defect which secondarily leads to the cerebral symptomatology?

The general evidence would seem to indicate that the liver has nothing to do with the cerebral troubles until the liver itself fails and then the same mechanisms as would operate in the production of hepatic coma may come into action. In favor of this is the predominance of cerebral symptoms in the face of relatively mild hepatic symptoms. On the other hand the hepatic dysfunction may kill the patient before the lenticular difficulties set in. The so called "formes frustes" have been frequently observed in families with this disease and in which hepatic or cerebral symptoms may be present alone. Copper seems to be precipitated in many organs in Wilson's disease, e.g.: liver, brain, cornea, lens and skin. The exact role of the increased brain copper is not clear but such an excess can "poison" local cerebral enzyme systems. Parallel lenticular lesions have been known for years as a result of manganese and cyanide poisonings where again enzymatic inactivation is the best explanation. Further study of the cerebral biochemical features is necessary before one can draw any sweeping conclusions.

Coke and Shaw (283) described a case of hepatolenticular degeneration in a man with chronic heart disease, liver infection and alcoholism. This was considered to be an acquired case of Wilson's disease and Kayser-Fleischer corneal rings were not present nor was there any deposition of copper in the liver or brain. The authors considered hypoglycemia as a cause in this particular instance and further suggested that there are a group of conditions which make up the hepatolenticular syndrome. Without the biochemical criteria or familial features cases like this should not be classified under the eponym of Wilson's disease and would better be classified under hepatoencephalomyelopathy.

Treatment

The use of BAL (British Anti-Lewisite-dimethylcaprol) by Cumings (55) in 1951 offered some hope to the treatment of this condition. Since then many cases have been helped by the use of this compound. Although the improvement lasts only as long as the BAL is given, and while it increases the urinary copper excretion it does not cure the disease and does not influence the aminoaciduria. Warnock and Neill (277) described a case of Wilson's disease in a young male of 16 who had hepatomegaly at age 3, Kayser-Fleischer rings at 10 and later ascites, edema, and jaundice with hypercupruria. With the administration of BAL the hepatic dysfunction disappeared and the nerological symptoms remained absent. Hornbostel (254) described 2 cases of hepatolenticular degeneration treated with BAL which caused an increase in urinary copper excretion, improvement of neurologic symptoms and cataract regression but which had no effect on the amino aciduria or the serum copper. Cumings (55), in 1951, and

Denny-Brown and Porter (271), in same year, reported on the successful treatment of this disease in 4 and 5 cases, respectively. In 1 case treated by the author, BAL resulted in considerable clinical improvement but relapses occurred when the treatment was stopped. Bearn (280) observed improvement of neurological symptoms in some cases treated with BAL but could not demonstrate improvement in the hepatic symptomatology. From such conflicting reports it would seem that BAL is only effective in causing clinical benefit at some time prior to the development of permanent tissue changes. The yardstick to be used in determin-

Mechanism of Action of BAL and Copper

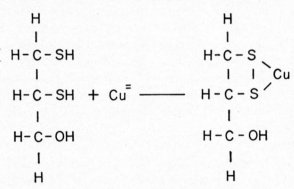

Fig. 12. Mechanism of Action of BAL.

ing this point is not clear. Its chief value would seem to be in the early case.

BAL is not efficient in so far as the removal of copper is concerned. It has a molecular weight of 124 and, if it removed 1 atom of copper with an atomic weight of 63, a 200 milligram dose of BAL should combine with and remove 100 milligrams of copper. In actual practice this dosage results in the removal of about 1 milligram of copper. Nevertheless it should be tried and a suitable course is 1.5 cubic centimeters of a 10 per cent solution of BAL in peanut oil intramuscularly, two to four times a day for 10 to 14 days. Local abscess formations are troublesome. The mode of action of this chelating agent is as shown in Figure 12.

Other chelating agents such as sodium versenate have been used with some successes. Cohen (284) reported on the successful use of an atropine like compound related to artane (1-phenyl-1-cyclopentl-3 piperidine-1-propanal hydrochloride).

Walshe (285, 286) has recently studied the use of penicillamine (dimethylcystine) in Wilson's disease. This compound has been demonstrated in the urine of patients with liver injury who received parenteral penicillin. Because of its solubility, rapid renal excretion and stability it was tried in this disease to promote copper excretion. Six cases previously reported by Denny-Brown and others were treated with 0.5 to 1.5 grams per day. The drug was shown to be more effective in the excretion of copper than was BAL. There were no side effects. Further clinical trials are awaited. Other sulfur containing compounds including methionine, 4-beta-tetramethylcystine have been tested and shown to be ineffective in promoting copper excretion suggesting that the SH group alone is not the key factor but that the SH ring structure is the effective part. Corticoids have been used but have not proved particularly beneficial in this disease.

The relationship of the aberrant copper metabolism to the aminoaciduria and of both to the production of cerebral symptoms remains to be clarified. The evidence seems to indicate that a defect in copper metabolism is the important factor and that in the brain and liver it is independently precipitated producing symptoms referable to each organ. The precipitation of copper in other tissues accounts for some of the other signs observed in this disease. The exact explanation of the cerebral symptoms and the exact nature of the copper defect are yet to be answered.

Chapter IX

PATHOLOGICAL ASPECTS

A PATHOLOGICAL evaluation of the brain is both important and necessary to an understanding of liver brain relationships. Its importance is somewhat diminished now in light of recent work and will continue to decline for it is apparent that light microscopy used chiefly in descriptive pathology and microscopic anatomy has reached its peak and has little more to offer as an investigative weapon in this particular disorder. Virtually nothing has been added of any significance by this instrument in the past 40 years as all changes now regarded as important were known and described 40 or more years ago. The preparation of the specimen with fixatives, dyes, and alcohols removes and alters neuronal structures and membrane characteristics so that the living state is far from what is visualized on the finished slide. Electron microscopy will doubtless provide more detailed information but is at the moment also subject to the same fixation artefacts of shrinkage and distortion.

While there have been many accounts of the cerebral changes in hepatic disease, most studies have embraced but a small number of cases and few attempts have been made to grade cerebral changes or to correlate the changes with the pathology in the liver or with liver function studies. Cerebral pathology will be considered under the following headings: (1) historical review; (2) case material; (3) complicating factors (post-mortem autolysis, cerebrovascular disease, terminal diseases); (4) gross changes; (5) microscopic study: (a) nerve cell changes; (b) myelin changes; (c) glial changes; (6) the spinal cord; (7) discussion and conclusion; (8) relation between neuropathological changes and liver function tests.

HISTORICAL REVIEW

Although macroscopic and microscopic cerebral changes have been observed in hepatic disease they are neither constant nor pathognomonic. Both early and recent authors remarked upon the discrepancy between the clinical findings and the lack of change at autopsy. While most pathological studies have been on Wilson's disease relatively few have stressed cerebral alterations in other hepatic diseases and much disagreement exists as to the relative importance of the microscopic changes.

Gross lesions of the brain were not observed in the cases of hepatic coma reported by Frerichs (11), Bright (9), and Budd (10). Gowers (15-17), Homen (18), Ormerod (19), Westphal (13), Strümpell (21), and Wilson (26) later reported on gross cavitation of the putamen, caudate nucleus and globus pallidus in hepatolenticular degeneration. According to Wilson, gross changes were also noted in the ansa lenticularis, corpus Luysii, Forel's bundle, the striothalamic and striosubthalamic fiber tracts. Greenfield, Poynton and Walsh (29), in 1924, noted gross atrophy of the corpus striatum with minimal involvement of the globus pallidus in a case of Wilson's disease. Although Wilson stressed gross changes in the basal ganglionic region, macroscopic lesions have been found in other parts of the brain. Barnes and Hurst (35), Bielschowsky and Hallervorden (110), Ostertog (287), von Braunmuhl (288), Hamburger and Kozol (253) observed convolutional necrosis in hepato-lenticular degeneration. Richter (289), in 1948, reported a similar case with severe necrosis and atrophy of the frontal cortex.

Greater emphasis was placed on the microscopic changes in the brain as a result of the publication of Hösslin and Alzheimer (31), in 1912. They describe an irregular lobulated cell, larger than the normal astrocyte, having scant cytoplasm, a few condensed threads of chromatin, a large dark staining nucleolus which has become known as the Alzheimer cell. These cells were found in many parts of the brain and were considered at the time to be characteristic of pseudosclerosis. Similar cells were observed in Wilson's disease by Spielmeyer (37), in 1920, and he commented on the close resemblance to neurones primarily because of the intense staining nucleolus. Spielmeyer demonstrated that Wilson's disease and pseudosclerosis had identical microscopic and gross changes. That this cell was not present in all cases of Wilson's disease was illustrated by the reports of Barnes and Hurst, in 1925 (35) and 1929 (36), in which Alzheimer's cells were found in only two of four members of a family with this disorder.

Widespread cerebral changes were reported by Boenheim (101), Bielschowsky and Hallervorden (110) including astrocytic proliferation, diffuse demyelination, neuronophagia and non-specific nerve cell changes. Von Braunmuhl (288) observed gliosis, oligodendrogliosis and perivascular demyelination and severe ganglion cell changes. Jervis, Notkin, Freiman and Moore (290) found chronic nerve cell changes, satellitosis and gitter cells in addition to glial, myelin changes, and abundant Alzheimer cells in the cortex, dentate nucleus and olives.

Leigh and Card (106), in 1949, reported on degeneration of the posterior and lateral columns of the spinal cord in a case of hepato-lenticular degeneration and Gysin and Cooke (64), in 1950, commented upon the marked ferrugination and calcification of blood vessels in the same disease.

From these few reports it is evident that the cerebral alterations in Wilson's diseases are much more extensive than the title would suggest.

Alterations similar to those observed in Wilson's disease have been found in patients with a wide variety of hepatic diseases. Crandall and Weil (79), in 1933, pointed out the similarities between the cerebral lesions in humans and experimental animals with hepatic disease. Scherer (291), in 1933, studied 41 cases of varied liver pathology and demonstrated Alzheimer cells in 90 per cent of his cases. Stadler (282), in 1935, and Adams and Davidson (292), in 1949, agreed that this cell was the most characteristic feature of the brain pathology in hepatic disease. Alexander (293), in 1942, noted cerebral changes which were identical with Wilson's disease in a case of alcoholic cirrhosis and Waggoner and Malamud (48), in 1942, reported cerebral changes identical with those of hepato-lenticular degeneration in five cases of varied hepatic pathology.

Weinstein and Davidson (177), in 1946, reported on arteriolar thrombosis, pervascular demyelination and microglial proliferation in hepatitis. Baker (105), in 1949, noted widespread nerve cell changes in 8 of 18 cases with diverse liver pathology but emphasized perivascular and diffuse demyelination as being more characteristic of hepatic disease.

It is evident from this review that any part of the nervous system may be involved in hepatic disease and that the underlying hepatic pathology may be quite diverse.

CASE MATERIAL

The present study consists of a histological examination of the brain in 42 cases of hepatic insufficiency and coma. In all cases, complete post mortem examination was made with the exception of the spinal cord which was removed in only 5 instances. The peripheral nerves were not examined in any case and it is doubtful if an evaluation of that part of the nervous system would be fruitful since no symptoms have been recorded referable to it. The brain at autopsy was removed by the usual method and placed in 10 per cent formalin. After 7 to 10 days of fixation the brain was examined grossly and cut. Sections were made from the following locations; frontal, parietal, temporal, occipital cortexes, basal ganglia, midbrain, pons, medulla and cerebellum. In most instances 10 to 15 blocks of tissue were taken from each brain for microscopic study. The tissues were stained by hematoxylin and eosin and Nissl and Weil techniques used for neuronal and myelin changes, respectively. Special stains such as the van Giesson elastic tissue stain, the Perl stain for iron and the Holzer stain for glia were used when indicated.

The case material has been discussed in Chapter III. Although cirrhosis was the most frequent liver condition underlying the coma, less than half of the cases were of this type of hepatic disease. This differs from most reports which show a much greater percentage of cirrhosis. A better evaluation of other hepatic diseases, however, is possible.

Age

Mention has been made of age factors in this group of patients and is mentioned here again. Hepatic disease in general is more often associated with adulthood than childhood and is more frequent in the fourth, fifth and sixth decades. The average age of the adults in this study was 55.7 years. Five children are included with ages ranging from infancy to 9 years. Extremes in age introduce different factors which must be accounted for in the final interpretation. In the case of the infants, the cerebral metabolism differs from the adult, myelination is not complete and the cells are more immature. On the other hand advancing age produces changes in the central nervous system which must be interpolated in the final analysis of pathologic change.

It will be seen later that severe cerebral changes occur in the young as well as the older brain. It can be said in general that the clinical and pathological changes are of equal or greater magnitude in the child than in the adult. Spence and Ogilvie (171), Snell and Butt (99), Murphy, Chalmers, Eckhardt and Davidson (144), and Walshe (61) have expressed the same opinion. From this it might appear that the age factor cannot be too important despite the opinion of Crandall and Weil (79), that the combination of chronic hepatic disease and arteriosclerosis makes conclusions as to the histopathological changes in the central nervous system impossible.

Sex

In this series there were 16 females and 26 males. Most statistical studies of hepatic disease show a more uniform distribution as cirrhosis is generally considered to be more common in males and infections of the liver more frequent in females. Little significance can be attached to this factor in so far as changes in the nervous system are concerned.

COMPLICATING FACTORS

A critique of this nature necessitates consideration of all factors which would enter into and complicate the interpretation of microscopic changes in the nervous system. In dealing with human beings there are always many variables which while they cannot be eradicated must be considered. Sclerosis of the cerebral vessels, post-mortem autolysis and concurrent and terminal diseases are such complicating factors. Allusion has already been made to age factors.

Post-mortem Changes

Autolytic changes in the central nervous system are always present to a greater or lesser extent in human material and many pathological changes can be produced by technical procedures.

In 1897, Neppi (294) studied and observed changes in the anterior horn cells in dogs within 48 hours after death and concluded that such changes occurred late. Barabacci and Campacci (295) in the same year found changes 3 hours after death. More recently Koenig and Koenig (296), in 1952, in a well controlled study showed post-mortem changes in the ventral horn cells within half an hour of death. Autolytic changes of this type are sometimes indistinguishable from those changes occurring as a result of acute infections or toxic conditions. Jungman and Kimmelstiel (297) showed how rapidly biochemical changes occur following death. Within one-half hour there is a maximum increase in the lactic acid concentration, phosphocreatine is hydrolyzed and adenosine triphosphate decomposed in 30 minutes according to Weil (298). This would affect the staining of the cell.

The "chronic nerve cell disease" of Nissl is characterized by cell shrinkage, dark stained cytoplasm, tortuous dendrites and hyperchromatic nucleus. Similar, if not identical, changes can be produced as a result of fixation. Immersion fixed brains within a few minutes of removal from freshly killed animals showed greater changes than perfused specimens. The appearance of chronic nerve cell disease is due in part to the hypertonicity of the fixing fluid which by osmosis causes loss of cell fluid, condensation of the Nissl with subsequent appearance of deep staining. Weil (298) cautions against evaluating ganglion cell changes in conditions in which the fluids of the nervous system contain toxic substances as in uraemia, hepatic disease and septicaemia. In 1932, Quastel and Wheatley (299) wrote that "hardening a tissue in alcohol or treatment with the usual fixing agents produces changes in the tissue constituents which are greater than would ever be supposed to occur when in the living condition."

However, while the post-mortem changes are to be considered in the pathological interpretation, they cannot be the sole cause for if such were the case, all cells might be expected to exhibit the same type of alteration. Furthermore, post-mortem changes in addition to affecting the neurones are also accompanied by other changes such as swelling of the oligodendroglia and widened perivascular spaces. Significant post-mortem changes do not occur in the nucleus until 24 hours after death of the tissue.

Only one brain was fixed by perfusion. The average elapsed time between post mortem and tissue death was 4.6 hours with a range of from 1 to 15 hours. The time could not be determined in 6 cases. While the amount of time elapsed is not undue in consideration of autopsy technical standards in this country, nevertheless considerable chemical alteration in the cells takes place and interpretation of the nerve cell alterations must be done with care.

Terminal and Concurrent Diseases

Another factor to be considered is the presence of other diseases whether terminal, pre-existing or clinically asymptomatic and found only at autopsy. In order to evaluate the effect of such factors the case material was carefully examined for mention of significant pre-existing diseases and for the presence of terminal infections. Table XXI is an analysis of such data. Column two represents the pathological diagnosis of the hepatic lesion, and all other conditions are included under the term secondary diagnoses (column three).

Pulmonary infections were found at autopsy in 14 cases. All of these were considered as terminal and there was no clinical evidence of pulmonary lesion in any of the cases. In most instances the pulmonary lesion was a bronchopneumonia confined to the lower lobes or was a purulent bronchitis. The latter was observed in 4 cases. The leucocytosis found in 15 cases may be due

TABLE XXI

PRIMARY HEPATIC PATHOLOGY AND COMPLICATING PATHOLOGY FOUND AT AUTOPSY

Case Ref. No.	Etiology of Hepatic Insufficiency	Secondary Pathologic Diagnosis
1	Obstructive cirrhosis	———
2	Obstructive cirrhosis	bronchitis, terminal
3	Subacute yellow atrophy	———
4	Obstructive cirrhosis	pneumonia, terminal
5	Subacute yellow atrophy	duodenal ulcer, mild
		pyelonephritis, arteriosclerosis
6	Subacute yellow atrophy	arthritis
		pneumonia, terminal
7	Portal cirrhosis	bronchopneumonia, mild
8	Hepatitis, serum	purulent bronchitis
9	Portal cirrhosis (alcohol)	general arteriosclerosis
		mild coronary sclerosis
		hemolytic anaemia
10	Portal cirrhosis	ulcer, duodenal
		lobar pneumonia
11	Obstructive cirrhosis	carcinoma pancreas
		purulent bronchopneumonia
12	Subacute yellow atrophy	———
13	Portal cirrhosis (alcohol)	———
14	Obstructive cirrhosis	pneumonia, terminal
15	Portal cirrhosis	———
16	Acute yellow atrophy	cerebral arteriosclerosis
		bronchopneumonia, terminal
17	Obstructive cirrhosis	cerebral sclerosis
		mild arteriosclerotic heart
18	Portal cirrhosis-F. deg. (alcohol)	anaemia
19	Portal cirrhosis (alcohol)	coronary sclerosis
20	Portal cirrhosis-F. deg. (alcohol)	bronchopneumonia, mild
21	Hepatitis	———
22	Portal cirrhosis (alcohol)	———
23	Portal cirrhosis	pulmonary congestion
24	Portal cirrhosis (alcohol)	moderate coronary sclerosis
		bronchopneumonia
		G.I. hemorrhage
25	Abscess	mild coronary sclerosis
26	Metastatic melanoma	pulmonary oedema
27	Hepatic necrosis	———
28	Portal cirrhosis	pulmonary atelectasis
29	Obstructive	nephritis, interstitial
		atelectasis
30	Hepatitis, recurrent	massive G.I. hemorrhage
31	Hepatitis	pneumonia, terminal, mild

TABLE XXI—(*continued*)

Case Ref. No.	Etiology of Hepatic Insufficiency	Secondary Pathologic Diagnosis
32	Hemochromatosis	————
33	Portal cirrhosis (alcohol)	————
34	Portal cirrhosis	hypertension coronary sclerosis
35	Obstructive cirrhosis	————
36	Acute yellow atrophy	coronary sclerosis, mild
37	Acute yellow atrophy	————
38	Subacute yellow atrophy	cerebral arteriosclerosis coronary sclerosis with myocardial infarction
39	Metastatic carcinoma	————
40	Portal cirrhosis (alcohol)	glomerulonephritis, chronic inactive valvulitis severe pneumonia
41	Amyloidosis	cardiac hypertrophy
42	Fatty degeneration	purulent bronchitis

in part to the pulmonary pathology which in general was described as mild and in one case as severe.

Generalized arteriosclerosis was found in a sufficient degree to be mentioned in autopsy protocols. Sclerosis of the coronary vessels was noted in 7 cases and in most instances was mild. A healed posterior myocardial infarct was noted in 1 patient.

Anaemia was mentioned at autopsy in 3 cases, although clinically it was found in 47 per cent of the cases.

A search of the records for previous disease yielded only the 2 cases of ulcerative colitis. One patient had hypertension for 6 years (Case 41) but this was asymptomatic. An abnormal bleeding tendency for 18 years was noted by the patient with amyloidosis (Case 42). Complicating conditions were absent in 10 cases.

While the majority of the case material exhibited some additional pathologic state at autopsy, in most instances it was terminal and of a mild degree. The presence of these conditions is to be reckoned with in general for in no case can it be presumed that the secondary diagnosis was the sole cause of the cerebral change. The part played by the secondary conditions is impossible to evaluate.

Cerebrovascular Sclerosis

Weil expressed the opinion that changes in the central nervous system in hepatic disease are impossible to interpret because of the associated disease of the cerebral blood vessels. Wilens (300) has shown that there is no significant difference in the extent of atherosclerosis in cirrhotics as compared with other individuals of comparable status, age and sex. In this study the cerebral blood vessels were considered normal in 23 or 54 per cent of the cases (Table XXII). The remaining 19 cases showed varying degrees of

TABLE XXII

RELATIVE FREQUENCY OF PATHOLOGY IN THE CEREBRAL BLOOD VESSELS

Pathological State	Number of Cases	Per Cent of Cases
Normal	23	54
Slight sclerosis	12	28
Moderate sclerosis	5	11
Severe sclerosis	2	4

vascular change ranging from mild sclerosis to severe sclerosis with calcification of blood vessel walls. While it is true that cerebral vessel sclerosis is sometimes associated with indefinite and diffuse changes including mild forms of cell ischaemia, demyelination and cavity formation, such changes may be present in a clinically intact individual and their presence be uncovered only at post-mortem examination. Changes of the above nature are themselves to be considered with caution as an index of cerebral dysfunction. It is highly unlikely that changes associated with cerebral arteriosclerosis as described above and even those more advanced will produce intermittent and prolonged coma. The effect of the sclerosed blood vessels on myelin and ganglion cell changes is shown in Table XXIII. The gradation of cerebral lesions will be outlined in the section on microscopic changes.

It is apparent from this table that sclerosed blood vessels were no more productive of alterations in the neurones or myelin than normal cerebral vessels. Further evidence of this is found in the cases of children in whom the cerebral vessels are normal whereas

TABLE XXIII

FREQUENCY OF CEREBRAL CHANGES WITH NORMAL AND ABNORMAL
CEREBRAL BLOOD VESSELS

Location of Alteration	Grade	Blood Vessels Number of Cases	
		Normal	Sclerosed (all degrees)
Neuronal cortex	1	6	3
	2	10	11
	3	7	3
Basal gang.	1	8	5
	2	8	8
	3	8	6
Myelin cortex	1	6	6
Diffuse	2	12	6
	3	1	2
Perivascular	1	5	5
	2	6	1
	3	1	2
Basal gang.	1	4	2
Diffuse	2	3	5
	3	1	1
Perivascular	1	6	2
	2	3	1
	3	1	2

the myeline and neuronal changes are quite severe. The over all effect of the vascular change on the production of cerebral alterations is most difficult to evaluate but for the reasons given here it would appear to be minimal.

GROSS ALTERATIONS

In this series of cases no gross abnormalities were observed except for the mention of arteriosclerotic plaques around the basal cerebral vessels. In one case a small meningioma was found over the vertex and had nothing to do with the clinical symptomatology.

MICROSCOPIC CHANGES

Nerve Cell Changes (Figs 13-16)

Changes in the cellular morphology and staining reactions were observed in both neurones and in supporting elements. It could be

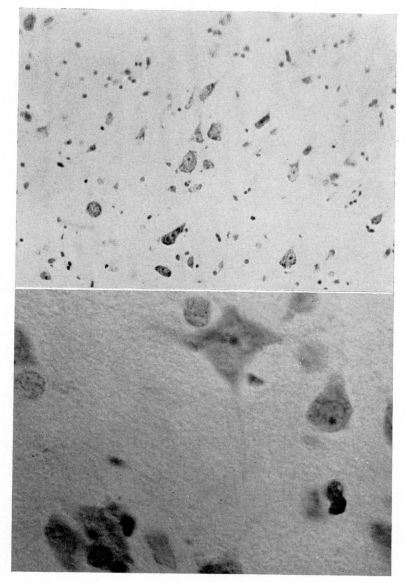

Fig. 13. Perinuclear chromatolysis in cortical neurones. This type of change is found in many toxi-infectious states and is not characteristic of hepatic encephalopathy.

Fig. 14. High power magnification of cortical neurones further showing non-specific cellular change. Cytoplasmic vacuoles are present in cell on the right.

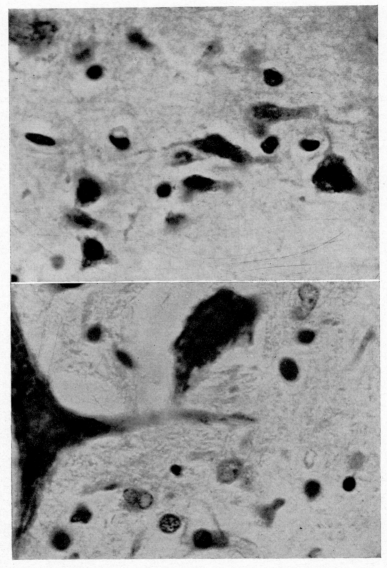

FIG. 15. Chronic nerve cell changes showing hyperchromatic and pyknotic cells.

FIG. 16. Hyperchromatic neurones with normally located Nissl substance and some cell shrinkage. Changes of this type are readily reproducible by fixatives. An Alzheimer cell is to be seen in the upper right corner.

stated at the outset that the changes to be described could occur as a result of complicating factors such as post-mortem techniques, terminal diseases, and alteration in the cerebral vessels. It was pointed out, however, that none of those factors in itself could produce the changes noted nor account for the clinical symptomatology. Recognizing both the difficulties in assessing neuronal changes and the drawbacks to any system of classification, it was felt that if any value, whether positive or negative, were to accrue from a study of neurones, a system of gradation would be necessary. Otherwise, the terms "mild" and "severe" would be used and of which there is considerable latitude of interpretation. In general, neuronal changes are considered as either acute or chronic. In this study two types of nerve cell alteration were observed. The first or acute change is characterized by swelling, chromatolysis of Nissl substance, fragmentation of processes and loss of staining properties. Ghost cells, eccentricity of nucleus and vacuolated cytoplasm were considered as more advanced stages of the acute process or perhaps as a subacute process. Chronic nerve cell change consisting of shrinkage and distortion of cell body, tortuosity of processes, pyknosis of the nucleus with deep staining was the second type noted. Both acute and chronic nerve cell alterations were noted to some extent in all cases. No attempt is made to determine the predominance of acute or chronic changes in this case material. The classification used here is based on the over all number and percentage of abnormal ganglion cells whether acute or chronic in comparison to normal cells in the same area. Except initially when cell counts were made on several areas to establish a baseline, an estimation of abnormal cells was done. The over all change was assessed for each brain and graded as to severity as follows: grade 1 or mild, representing 10 to 20 per cent of the cells damaged, grade 2 or moderate, representing damage to 30 to 50 per cent of the neurones and grade 3 or severe in which 60 per cent or more of the neurones were altered. While such a grading system admittedly has drawbacks and is subject to the same criticism of any similar system of gradation, it nevertheless provides some basis for evaluating the cerebral changes.

The frequency of graded nerve cell change in the cortex of

TABLE XXIV

FREQUENCY OF GRADED CORTICAL NEURONAL CHANGES

Gradation	Number of Cases	Per Cent of Cases
Grade 1, mild	9	21
Grade 2, moderate	22	52
Grade 3, severe	11	26

this case material is shown in Table XXIV. Examination of this table shows that mild involvement was present in 9 cases or 21 per cent, moderate or grade 2 alterations were most frequent and present in 22 cases or 52 per cent, while grade 3 or more severe cerebral involvement was evident in only 11 instances or 26 per cent of the cases.

The predominance of striatal symptomatology in Wilson's disease and the relative frequency of striatal symptoms in other forms of acquired liver disease suggests a susceptibility of this part of the central nervous system to the effects of a damaged liver. Similarly, pathological lesions in this area of the brain have been severe and frequently encountered. Using the same criteria described above, mild changes or grade 1 were found in 30 per cent of the cases; These values are shown in Table XXV. Comparison of these figures with alterations in the cortical neurones demonstrates a more uniform distribution of all three grades in the basal ganglia. Mild and severe changes were more frequently noted and moderate changes less frequently found. There would seem to be somewhat more severe involvement of the basal ganglia in so far as nerve cell changes are concerned.

Brain Stem and Cerebellum. No significant nerve cell changes were noted in the brain stem or cerebellum except in Cases 2 and

TABLE XXV

RELATIVE FREQUENCY OF NEURONAL CHANGES IN THE BASAL GANGLIA

Gradation	Number of Cases	Per Cent of Cases
Grade 1, mild	13	30
Grade 1, moderate	16	38
Grade 3, severe	13	30

3 in which severe nerve cell changes were observed in the pons and medulla.

Discussion of Neuronal Changes. It is apparent from the foregoing that it is impossible to draw any conclusions as to whether or not the observed neuronal changes were secondary to the hepatic disease. Cell changes similar to those seen in acute and chronic states can be found in small numbers in the normal brain. Post-mortem autolysis and fixation are capable of causing similar changes. The role of vascular disease and terminal infections is difficult to assess and further complicates the interpretation. Similar opinions have been expressed by Wilson (27), Quastel and Wheatley (299), Walshe (61) and Bielschowsky and Hallervorden (110) who recorded severe neuronal changes. Wilson noted some tigrolysis and pigmentary degeneration but regarded that as too slight to be of any significance.

On the whole neuronal changes must be regarded as nonspecific and not severe. The only proper conclusion is that the observed neuronal changes are the net result of hepatic disease, post mortem autolysis, tissue preparation techniques and terminal infections.

Myelin Alterations (Figs. 17-22)

Like the neurones of the central nervous system the myelin sheaths are subject to the effects of the post-mortem period and fixation. The structure described as the myelin sheath in formalin fixed material is but a distorted image of the original. Fixatives such as formalin are hydrolysates and coagulators. Alcohol and xylol are both fat solvents. Weil (301), in 1929, showed that the increase in the acidity of the fixing fluid parallels an increase in water soluble phosphorous compounds and a decrease in phospholipids that can be extracted from the fixing fluid. The galactolipids which make up a large portion of myelin are more resistant to the effects of formalin. Formalin alters the solubility of lipids, reducing the ability to extract such substances by ether or alcohol.

Despite the role of fixation techniques alterations of the myelin when present are fairly reliable as an index of some cerebral dysfunction. In this study changes in the myelin were of either a

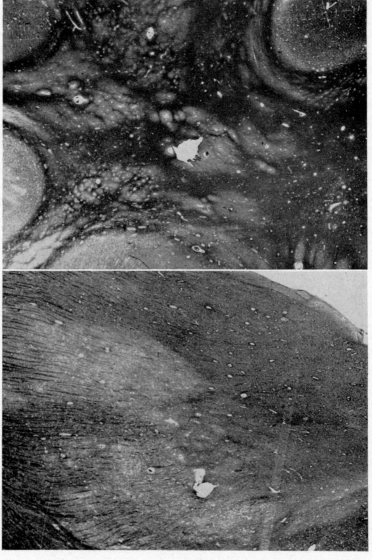

Fig. 17. Mottled appearance of demyelinated areas in white substance.
Fig. 18. Diffuse demyelination in basal ganglia.

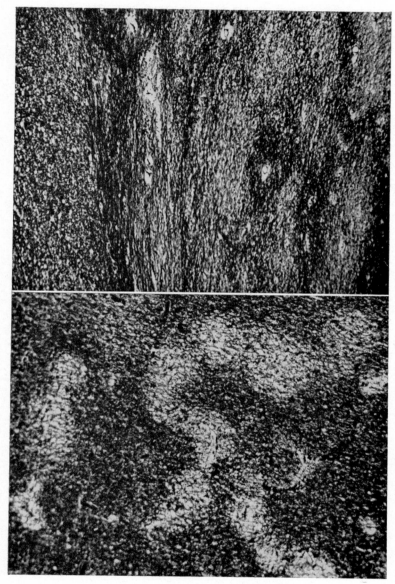

Fɪɢ. 19. Diffuse demyelination.
Fɪɢ. 20. Higher power of perivascular demyelination.

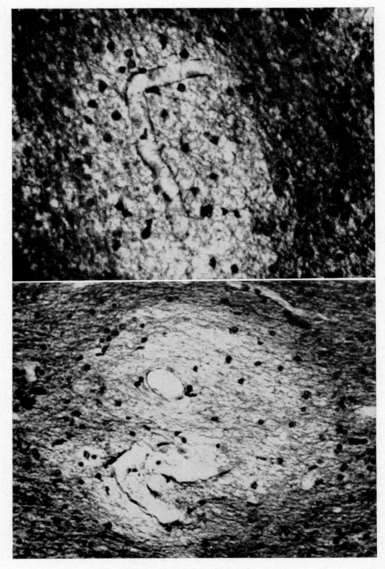

Fig. 21. Perivascular demyelinization.
Fig. 22. Perivascular demyelinization.

TABLE XXVI

PERCENTAGE OF MYELIN CHANGE IN CASE MATERIAL

	Number of Cases	*Per Cent of Cases*
Myelin change, all types	36	85
No myelin change	6	15

diffuse, patchy or perivascular pattern. The latter frequently merged imperceptibly into large areas of diffuse demyelination.

A system of gradation was again considered necessary to evaluate the myelin changes properly. The gradation was based upon the observed frequency of demyelination on a low power field whether perivascular or diffuse. Grade 1, or mild change, represented 1 area of perivascular demyelination or 1 area of diffuse demyelination per low power field. Grade 2, or moderate involvement, represented 2 areas of perivascular change and diffuse demyelination per low power field. Grade 3, or severe change, is defined as 3 or more areas of perivascular alteration and large zones of diffuse demyelination. Table XXVI shows the over-all frequency of the various grades of myelin change. This table shows that 85 per cent of the cases had myelin changes of some variety and degree. Six cases or 15 per cent had no alterations of the myelin.

The frequency and severity of demyelination exclusive of the basal ganglionic regions is shown in Tables XXVII and XXVIII from which it is shown that diffuse demyelination is more frequent than the perivascular form. Only 3 cases had severe demyelination. Of the 3 cases one was a child of 8 months who had

TABLE XXVII

FREQUENCY OF MYELIN CHANGE EXCLUSIVE OF THE BASAL GANGLIA

Type of Change	*Number of Cases*	*Per Cent of Cases*
Diffuse demyelination	33	78
Perivascular demyelination	20	47
Total No. with both types of change	34	80
No Myelin changes	8	19

TABLE XXVIII

FREQUENCY OF GRADED MYELIN CHANGE EXCLUDING THE BASAL GANGLIA

| | Demyelination | | | |
| | Perivascular | | Diffuse | |
	Number of Cases	Per Cent of Cases	Number of Cases	Per Cent of Cases
Grade 1	10	50	11	33
Grade 2	7	35	19	57
Grade 3	3	15	3	9
	20		33	

a congenital atresia of the bile duct with an obstructive type of cirrhosis. Of the remaining two, one was a woman of 53 who had acute yellow atrophy and the other a male of 62 with hemochromatosis. No complicating diseases were present with the exception of a mild degree of arteriosclerosis in the latter patient. On the other hand myelin alterations in the basal ganglia were less prominent and less severe as demonstrated in Tables XXIX and XXX. Both perivascular and diffuse demyelination are less frequent in the basal ganglia than in the rest of the brain as might be expected. The symptomatology from this region of the brain in this series of cases was not marked.

Discussion of Myelin Changes. Although myelin changes in general occurred less frequently than nerve cell changes their reliability as an index of cerebral pathology is somewhat greater. Diffuse demyelination was observed by Wilson (27), Von Braunmuhl (288), Bielschowsky and Hallervorden (110), Crandall and

TABLE XXIX

FREQUENCY OF MYELIN CHANGES UN BASAL GANGLIA

Type of Change	Number of Cases	Per Cent of Cases
Diffuse demyelination	15	37
Perivascular demyelination	16	38
Total No. (both types)	21	50
No myelin changes	21	50

TABLE XXX

FREQUENCY OF GRADED MYELIN CHANGE IN BASAL GANGLIA

| | *Demyelination* | | | |
| | *Perivascular* | | *Diffuse* | |
	Number of Cases	*Per Cent of Cases*	*Number of Cases*	*Per Cent of Cases*
Grade 1	9	55	8	42
Grade 2	4	25	9	47
Grade 3	3	18	2	10
	16		19	

Weil (79), Weinstein and Davison (177), Baker (105), Leigh and Card (106), Gysin and Cooke (64), Richter (289), Jervis, Notkin, Freiman and Moore (290). Perivascular myelin change has been emphasized by Baker (105). Von Braunmuhl (288), Crandall and Well (79), Weinstein and Davison (177) mentioned but did not stress perivascular lesions of this type.

The demyelination observed here was more striking in the white matter and inner cortical zones. The changes around some of the vessels were mild showing merely a fragmented, vacuolated distended appearance to the myelin. Around other vessels it was more complete. This process often extended some distance from the vessel and merged and coalesced into more diffuse myelin change. Fat granule cells were not noted except occasionally and neurones within the area showed some acute changes.

At this time it can be concluded that myelin alterations are present and that these changes occurred in 85 per cent of the cases which negates demyelination as the sole cause of coma since the latter occurred in almost 100 per cent of this case material. On the whole, myelin changes were much more striking than neuronal alterations.

Glial Changes (Figs. 23-26)

Since the publication of Hösslin and Alzheimer in 1912 in which glial changes were described in pseudosclerosis, many authors have regarded such a change as pathognomonic of hepatic disease. The outstanding feature of this change has been a cell known as the Alzheimer cell. Figure 23 is taken from the original work of Hösslin and Alzheimer. This type of cell was found in large numbers by Hösslin and Alzheimer, Spielmeyer (37), Stadler (282), Scherer (291), Adams, and Davidson (292), Waggoner and Malamud (48), von Braunmuhl (288), Bielschowsky and Hallervorden (110), Leigh and Card (106), Uzman and Brown (91), Richter (289), Ostertog (287), Jervis, Notkin, Freiman and Moore (290), Campbell and Morse (33), Barnes and Hurst (35), Green-

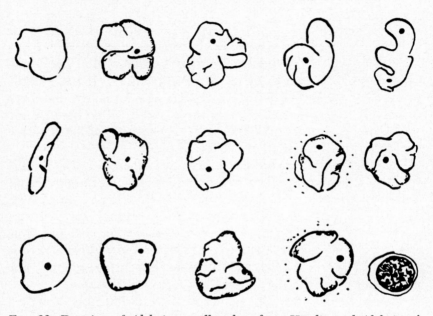

Fig. 23. Drawing of Alzheimer cells taken from Hösslin and Alzheimer's paper of 1912 showing variety of shapes taken by these cells.

field, Poynton and Walsh (29) and Inose (302). The cells are found in all parts of the central nervous system and with greater frequency in the basal ganglia, dentate nucleus and cerebellar folia. Adams believes the presence of such cells is so characteristic a feature that a diagnosis of hepatic encephalopathy cannot be made in their absence. Stadler (282) stated that over 90 per cent of the cases show this cell type.

Other glial alterations such as neuronophagia, gliosis, oligo-

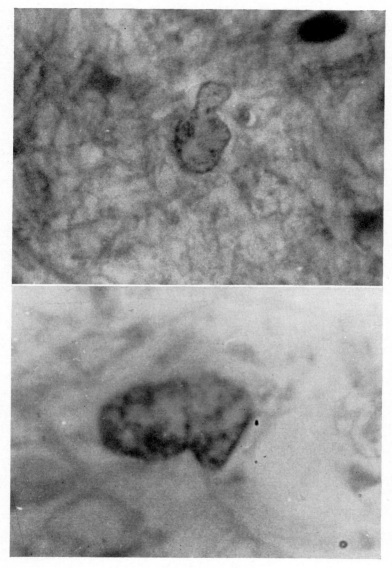

FIG. 24, 25. Alzheimer Cells.

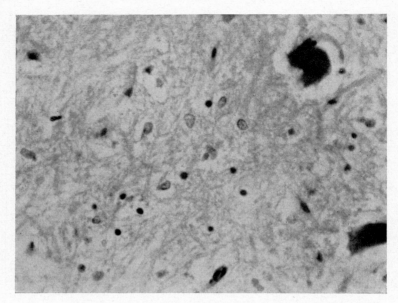

FIG. 26. Section through dentate nucleus showing a number
of Alzheimer cells.

dendrogliosis, gemistocytic astrocyte proliferation and compound
granular corpuscles have been noted. In this study, six types of
glial alteration were observed and these are listed in Table XXXI
with their relative frequency. No attempt is made to grade alterations of the glia.

It is evident from this table that the Alzheimer cell type was
the most frequently noted glial abnormality. This cell readily iden-

TABLE XXXI

FREQUENCY OF THE GLIAL CHANGES OBSERVED

Type of Change	Number of Cases	Per Cent of Cases
Alzheimer cells	22	52
Gliosis	13	30
Oligodendroglia swelling	5	11
Gemistocytes	4	9
Neuronophagia	3	7
Glial nodules	1	2

tifiable morphologically was found in all parts of the brain but with greater frequency in the dentate nucleus, cerebellar folia and basal ganglia. It was present in 22 cases or 52 per cent. In 3 cases such cells were found in the brain stem in large numbers. Although present in half of the cases, the cells were never found in such large numbers as described by Hösslin and Alzheimer (31), Stadler (282) and others.

Gliosis was observed in 13 cases or 30 per cent and in most instances was quite mild. There was no predilection for this change to occur in the basal ganglia or other regions of the brain.

Mild alterations of the oligodendroglia principally in the form of swelling were noted in 5 cases or 11 per cent. Oligodendroglia are sensitive to post-mortem autolysis under which circumstances the cell becomes swollen and its processes undergo clasmato-dendrosis. No particular significance is attached to this cellular alteration at the moment. Increased numbers of oligodendroglia were noted in several cases. Gysin and Cooke (64) reported an increase in this cell in their case as did Leigh and Card (106), Jervis, Notkin, Freiman and Moore (290), and von Braunmuhl (288).

Neuronophagia is frequently observed in infectious diseases and intoxications. Weil states that this represents an acute process and that the process or factor which initiates this change is quite obscure. Neuronophagia was present in 3 cases in a degree suffi-cient for mention. Similar alterations were reported by Crandall and Weil (79), Bielschowsky and Hallervorden (110) and von Braunmuhl (288).

Gemistocytic astrocytes were present in only 4 cases or 9 per cent. Glial nodules were present in one case. No particular sig-nificance can be attached to either of these changes because of their relative infrequent occurrence.

Discussion of Glial Changes. Considered as a whole the altera-tions of the glia demonstrated both regressive and reactive changes. The factors that cause pathologic changes in the neurones do not necessarily affect the glial elements. Intoxication and anaemia which may result in the death of a neurone, may how-ever, stimulate reactive changes in the glia. On the other hand, severe acute infectious involvement of the nervous system or even autolysis may cause regressive changes of glial cells. The oligodendroglia, because of their location around neurone, have been considered by some as lymphocytes. Their function is, however, much different. The accumulation around large neurones particularly in the deeper cortical layers giving the appearance of satellites, and along myelinated nerve fibers of the white matter indicates an intimate relation to nutrition according to some authors. The theory has been advanced that the oligodendroglia regulate the myelin formation of nerve sheaths and act as an intermediary in the exchange of metabolic products between neurones and brain fluids. Since the majority of glial changes observed in this study are found in many disease states, it is difficult to attach any real significance to them in an elucidation or cerebro-hepatic relationships.

The exception to this is the astrocytic alteration known as the Alzheimer cell. The factor that causes the transformation of the astrocyte to assume the morphological appearance described by Hösslin and Alzheimer is obscure. Campbell and Morse (33) felt the liver elaborated a toxin which acted on the glia producing this cell type. Stadler (303), in 1931, thought the Alzheimer cell might contain glycogen because he had observed glycogen rich cells in the liver of a similar appearance. This was disproved by Konowalow (304). Alexander (293), in 1942, noted Alzheimer cells in a variety of hepatic diseases and felt they are the same cell type as would be expected from necrosis due to deprivation and interference of the blood supply. Wood and Pendleton (305), in 1925, reported Alzheimer cells at autopsy in the brains of 14 Chinese observed during a famine in Shantung Province. Leigh and Card (106) suggested a dietary deficiency state also. They reported a case of hepato-lenticular degeneration with posterolateral column involvement and because of the picture of subacute combined degeneration of the cord, they drew a comparison between the Alzheimer cell and the megaloblastic response of the bone marrow in pernicious anaemia.

The Alzheimer cell was dismissed by Wilson as being neither constant nor specific. Siemerling and Jakob (306) noted them in infective cerebral states and in chronic epilepsy. They were not characteristic of the cases of Westphal (13), Schmidt (307), Kornyey (308), or Tschugunoff (309). They have been described in hepato-lenticular degeneration by Spielmeyer (37) and Pollack (39) and Barnes and Hurst (35). Campbell and Morse (33) in discussing the cells stated that the "polymorphous and ubiquitous glia which has been considered (wrongly) almost pathognomonic of pseudosclerosis is found in various toxic and infective processes although not in such abundance as in pseudosclerosis." Scharenberg and Brown (310) found only mild astroglial irritation in 3 cases of cirrhosis and inferred from this that the damage to the central nervous system in Laennec's cirrhosis is not identical with that in hepato-lenticular degeneration. Okinaka, Yashikawa, Toyoda, Mozai, Takayura and Kameyama (260) suggested that Alzheimer cells are formed as a result of damage by ingested copper.

To shed further light on the Alzheimer cell and because of the controversy, brains without liver disease were examined for Alzheimer cells. Morphologically identical cells were found in considerable numbers in the following conditions; erythroblastosis foetalis (premature), tuberous sclerosis, Alper's disease, Marie's cerebellar ataxia, paralysis agitans, Huntington's chorea, multiple sclerosis, Krabbe's disease, cerebral arteriosclerosis, cerebral contusion, the border zone of a glioblastoma multiforme and in two normal brains. While many of the above states may be deficiency states the ubiquity suggests that little stress should be placed on these cells as characteristic of hepatic disease. However, it can be said that the cells were observed in hepatic disease in greater numbers than in the above conditions but not in such abundant numbers as reported by other authors. With the exception of the Alzheimer cell, therefore, little significance can be accorded the glial alterations and which on the whole are not outstanding. Some of the alterations are reactive changes to neuronal degeneration whereas others are perhaps the result of the same factor that produced the neuronal and myelin changes while others are due to separate factors. The presence of the Alzheimer cell in 52 per cent of the cases is the outstanding glial alteration. Although the etiology of such a cellular change is obscure the presence of it in large numbers as reported by other authors and in one half of the cases in this study warrants some consideration. It is not to be considered, however, as a cerebral representative of hepatic disease only.

THE SPINAL CORD

Because of the preponderance of cerebral symptomatology in hepatic disease the spinal cord has been overlooked. Wilson (27) states the spinal cord is usually normal in lenticular degeneration. Von Braunmuhl (288) reported demyelination in the spinal cord and Leigh and Card (106) reported a case of hepato-lenticular degeneration associated with posterolateral column demyelination and gliosis. Although the cord was not examined, Gysin and Cooke (64) observed atrophy of scattered muscles in a case of hepato-lenticular degeneration suggesting spinal cord involvement.

In this series of 42 cases the spinal cord was examined in 5 instances. The anterior horn cells showed acute and chronic nerve cell changes in all cases along with neuronophagia. Demyelination of a mild degree in the lateral columns was observed in two cases. No clinical symptoms were reported in the cases with cord changes.

SUMMARY AND CONCLUSIONS OF CEREBRAL PATHOLOGIC STUDY

Alterations of neurones, myelin and glia were present in this study of 42 cases of hepatic disease. Nerve cell changes, graded on the basis of frequency of abnormality and noted in all cases, are not considered indicative of hepatic disease only. In 21 per cent, the changes were mild, in 52 per cent moderate, and in 26 per cent severe. Consideration in the interpretations of ganglion cell alterations must be given to the effects of autolysis and fixation and other complicating factors. Myelin changes were observed more frequently. Both perivascular and diffuse demyelination were present in this series and were less frequently observed in the basal ganglia. Severe demyelination was present in only 3 cases. Glial changes with the exception of the Alzheimer cell were not striking, and even the latter although present in 52 per cent of the cases was not found in copious numbers. Without doubt all changes described here contribute to the symptomatology of this group but the role played by each is impossible to determine.

Within the scope of present day techniques of tissue preparation, an evaluation of cerebral changes must be cautious. The general tone of this was aptly summed up by Wilson many years ago when he wrote "the attempt to use tissue reaction types as a means of dividing 'diseases' is one more example of a common fallacy that applies also to nerve cells; poisons and infections are endless but nerve and glial cells are severely restricted in their reactive possibilities. To assume that a particular type of reaction depends on a specific noza is a mistake."

RELATIONSHIP BETWEEN CEREBRAL CHANGES AND LIVER FUNCTION TESTS

Neuropathological changes of one type or other occurred in nearly every case of this study. The clinical symptomatology reflected this change and demonstrated the diffuseness of the cerebral alteration. In order to demonstrate whether or not a relationship exists between the liver function tests and cerebral changes the former were compared to the graded changes found in the neurones and myelin. No comparison with the glial alterations is attempted although in view of astrocytic changes such might be desirable. The changes in the glial elements, however, would contribute little to the general symptomatology of hepatic coma. This data is shown in Tables XXXII, XXXIII and XXXIV. There is a slight increase in the thymol turbidity, cephalin flocculation, and serum globulins as the cerebral neuronal changes become more severe. The bilirubin, although considerably elevated in all grades, nevertheless shows still greater elevation with more severe cerebral alterations. Grade 3 cerebral changes are accompanied by a considerable drop in hemoglobin as compared with Grade 1. No correlation existed with the urinary urobilinogen, porphyrins, serum cholesterol and alkaline phosphatase. The latter two were elevated only in 3 cases of obstructive jaundice.

TABLE XXXII

Showing Liver Function Data and Cerebral Changes

Case No.	Brain N.	Brain M.	Basal G. N	Basal G. M	TT	CC	Prothr. Time % of Normal	Alk. P'tase	Choles.	Esters	Hgb.	Urobilinogen U.	Bilirubin 1 min.	Bilirubin Tot.	Serum Prod. Tot.	Alb.	Glob.	Coproporphyrino
1	2	3	1	1	2	—	93	14.8	226	32	13.4	—	13.4	22.8	—	—	—	276
2	3	3	1	3	6	2—	100	46.8	536	31	10.3	—	9.5	8.2	—	1.8	5.2	—
3	3	3	3	3	10	4—	53	6.3	60	25	9.9	—	26.7	44.3	7.0	1.8	5.2	—
4	0	0	3	2	3	2—	73	65.8	154	20	10.6	EU 1.2	17.1	20.4	5.9	3.3	2.6	—
5	1	2	2	1	4	3—	63	.7	86	27	15.6		17.5	32.5	7.0	4.0	3.0	—
6	2	1	1	0	6	3—	36	42	96	31	11.2	mg/qd 38.7	14.0	28.9	5.8	2.6	3.2	—
7	2	1	1	0	4	2—	—	—	—	—	12.5		1.0	2.1	7.4	3.1	4.3	185
8	2	2	2	0	4.8	3—	19	5.2	76	22	12.8	mg/qd 2.2	4.6	8.7	7.0	3.8	3.2	218
9	3	1	3	0	9.5	4—	41	5.6	118	43	6.2	mg/qd 6.5	7.0	20.0	8.6	3.2	5.1	—
10	2	0	2	0	9.7	3—	—	—	—	—	13.2	mg/qd 67.2	.8	1.5	7.8	—	—	151
11	2	1	2	0	8.8	1—	58	17.9	650	32	12.7	12 EU/ 100 cc.	17.5	27.0	7.4	3.9	3.5	166
12	2	1	2	1	27.8	3—	44	8.3	164	6	10.0		19.0	27.7	8.5	2.3	6.2	—
13	1	2	2	0	6.1	4—	47	9.6	96	30	11.3	EU 3.6	4.6	11.1	7.5	2.5	5.0	174
14	2	1	2	0	4	2—	85	11.4	196	51	10.0		15.8	23.9	6.8	3.1	3.7	—
15	1	1	1	1	14.4	4—	—	—	—	—	11.9	EU			—	—	—	—
16	1	0	3	0			51	6.4	140	37	13.0		8.2	15.6	10.4	1.8	8.6	—
17	3	1	3	0			—	—	112	55	10.0	TR	5.6	11.6	4.5	2.4	2.1	—
18	3	0	3	0		3—	—	—	—	—	12.0		4—	2.2	—	—	—	—
19	2	2	2	1			55	—	—	—		31.0	.7		7.1	1.8	5.3	—
20	2	0	2	0	—	—	—	—	—	—			.5	1.8	—	—	—	—
21	2	0	2	0	1.0	2—	83	11	136	50	18.1		2.2	4.6	6.3	4.1	1.5	—
22	2	1	3	2	5	4—	68	7.6	148	55	11.0		1.5	3.7	6.5	2.1	4.4	280
23	2	2	1	0	0	0	40	8.3	74	—	12.0	4.3	23.7	45.9	—	—	—	288

TABLE XXXII—(continued)

Case No.	Brain N.	Brain M.	Basal G. N	Basal G. M	TT	CC	Prothr. Time % of Normal	Alk. P'tase	Choles.	Esters	Hgb.	Urobilinogen U.	Bilirubin 1 mm.	Bilirubin Tot.	Serum Prot. Tot.	Serum Prot. Alb.	Serum Prot. Glob.	Coproporphyrin
24	1	2	1	0	0	0	—	7.4	92	—	13.0	—	—	—	—	—	—	—
25	1	2	1	2	7	2—	114	—	204	52	11.0	10	15.1	30.4	5.9	2.7	3.2	—
26	1	2	1	2	7	—	100	—	256	46	14.0	—	4.8	7.7	5.5	3.0	2.5	—
27	2	2	2	2	4	4—	125	1.6	60	5	6.0	4 EU/100 cc.	11.5	18.7	6.3	1.9	4.4	—
28	3	2	3	2	—	4—	66	—	160	18	14.0	—	11.6	19.4	5.5	2.6	2.9	—
29	3	2	3	2	7	1—	80	6.4	228	—	11.0	—	23.2	33.6	5.0	2.0	3.0	140
30	3	2	2	0	15	3—	56	5.2	71	16	12.0	.6 mg/qd	13.5	17.7	5.8	1.4	4.4	—
31	3	0	3	0	—	—	54	—	166	73	7.0	—	4.5	8.1	6.6	3.3	3.3	—
32	3	3	2	1	—	0	109	—	27	13	15.0	7	.04	.5	6.6	3.7	2.9	737
33	3	2	3	1	4	4—	46	1.2	325	55	8.0	13	7.3	23.9	7.0	1.5	5.5	—
34	2	2	2	0	—	1—	92	6	325	68	14.0	3.9 EU	2.6	7.2	8.2	3.6	4.6	—
35	2	1	1	0	3	3—	—	23	—	—	14.0	1.2 EU/100 cc.	11.0	25.0	7.3	1.9	5.1	—
36	1	2	1	0	10	3—	—	—	205	68	14.0	—	8.6	15.7	8.9	3.8	5.1	300
37	3	2	3	2	11	3—	20	—	117	15	12.0	—	22.2	34.6	5.9	3.5	3.4	—
38	2	2	1	2	—	4—	50	—	—	—	—	—	4.5	15.0	5.1	1.2	3.9	—
39	2	0	2	0	—	—	120	—	—	42	7.0	—	—	25.0	6.4	2.7	3.7	—
40	2	2	1	2	6	4—	68	7.8	96	61	15.0	—	2.5	4.5	6.6	1.3	5.3	—
41	2	2	2	2	14	1—	55	7.8	169	63	7.0	5.4 EU	1.7	5.3	6.3	3.6	2.7	—
42	3	2	3	1	1	2—	88	7.1	—	—	12.0	—	4.8	8.7	3.9	1.8	2.1	—

N = Neuronal changes.
M = myelin changes.

TABLE XXXIII

AVERAGE VALUES OF LIVER FUNCTION TESTS COMPARED
TO NEURONAL CHANGES

| Neuronal Changes | TT | CC | Bilirubin | | Serum Prot. | | | Hgb. | Prothr. Time in % of Normal |
			1 min.	Tot.	Tot.	Alb.	Glob.		
Grade 1									
Cortex and white matter	5.4	2.0	8.8	16.4	7.4	2.7	4.1	13.2	90
Basal ganglia	6.2	2.5	9.3	17.8	7.2	2.7	5.0	11.6	81
Grade 2									
Cortex and white matter	7.5	2.8	8.6	16.6	6.8	2.8	3.9	11.1	66
Basal ganglia	8.7	2.8	8.2	14.4	6.8	2.9	3.4	15.1	66
Grade 3									
Cortex and white matter	7.9	3.0	11.0	19.7	5.8	2.3	3.5	9.8	56
Basal ganglia	6.3	3.1	11.6	20.7	6.0	2.4	3.6	10.4	58

A similar but less marked relationship holds for the myelin changes as shown in Table XXXIV. The flocculation tests show less variation than with neuronal changes. The prothrombin index is in the reverse relationship to that noted with the neuronal changes.

TABLE XXXIV

AVERAGE VALUES OF LIVER FUNCTION TESTS COMPARED
TO MYELIN CHANGES

| Myelin Changes | TT | CC | Bilirubin | | Serum Prot. | | | Hgb | Prothr. Time in % of Normal |
			1 min.	Tot.	Tot.	Alb.	Glob.		
Grade 1									
Cerebrum	9.4	3.3	8.2	16.3	7.7	2.3	5.4	10.8	47
Basal ganglia	6.4	3	11.5	21.7	6.2	2.5	3.7	12.0	67
Grade 2									
Cerebrum	6.8	2.6	11.3	20.1	6.3	2.7	3.5	12.0	69
Basal ganglia	7.1	3.2	11.1	18.5	5.9	2.5	3.3	10.8	71
Grade 3									
Cerebrum	8	2	18.1	21	6.8	2.7	4.0	11.7	87
Basal ganglia	8	3	18.1	21	6.8	2.7	4.0	11.7	87

Conclusions

No other conclusions can be drawn from such a study as this except to state that in general the more severe the hepatic disease the more abnormal the liver function tests and the more severe the cerebral changes. The inability to grade cerebral and hepatic lesions satisfactorily, the post mortem changes, and the time lapse between liver function studies and autopsy preclude any other conclusion. It is furthermore dangerous to relate the cerebral changes to any individual liver function tests. Although all of the tests are abnormal to some degree such a battery reflects only that liver function is impaired, a fact which can be as readily determined clinically by the presence of jaundice, ascites, and hepatomegaly. Hyperbilirubinemia, anaemia, elevated thymol turbidity, increased serum globulin, and a positive cephalin-flocculation were present in the majority of the cases. The degree of hepatic dysfunction cannot be ascertained by microscopic examination of the tissue and similarly the degree of cerebral involvement cannot be foretold by a study of liver function.

Chapter X

POSSIBILITIES, SPECULATIONS
AND CONCLUSIONS

T HE FRONTISPIECE to this monograph depicts the liver-brain relationship in the likeness of a tree, the roots of which are largely nourished by the liver and to a lesser extent other abdominal organs and the trunk of which conveys the hepatic metabolites to the brain. In our present stage of hepato-cerebral knowledge we are at the periphery of the tree, sampling the branches here and there. In this relationship we have but scratched the surface and have tended to forget that a combination of factors is more likely the cause of the cerebral manifestations than one substance alone.

Emphasis so far, has been placed upon the liver and its metabolites. We must now turn some attention to brain factors. As in the case of the chapter on the liver brevity is the keyword. There are several excellent books on brain chemistry to which the reader is referred for details (265, 311, 312). We are but at the beginning of this fascinating story. Electrophysiology of the brain is somewhat more advanced than cerebral biochemistry. The most frequently studied metabolic change in the brain has been that of oxygen consumption with somewhat less work done on glycolysis, amino acids, ammonia, lipids and proteins.

The metabolism of the brain is high and not only is there a difference in the metabolism between the central and peripheral nervous systems but considerable differences exist between cortex and white matter and the anterior and posterior parts of the brain. There is a very definite metabolic gradient from the frontal regions to the inferior brain areas. Because of this and because of the lack of oxidizing reserves in the brain, the forebrain structures may be decommissioned during low blood sugar and low oxygen levels while the medullary functions continue. The chief function of the cerebral metabolism during the resting state appears to be the maintenance of membrane integrity. When there is interference with cellular metabolism many biochemical changes occur among which is an egress of potassium ions and interruption of the resynthesis of creatine phosphate resulting in a change in membrane potential. Such alterations are not particularly specific to hepatic, renal or pancreatic disease but do indicate active rather than passive participation by the brain. Obviously not all cerebral changes can be accounted for by a fall in membrane potentials.

The resting and active metabolic states of the brain and the resting and active catalytic systems differ since the latter can be differentially inhibited. Furthermore the physiological response may be separated from changes in metabolism for a nerve may continue to conduct normally for many hours without increasing its oxygen consumption.

In a similar vein differences exist between parts of the neurones. The peripheral nerve has its own blood supply with various substrates and yet its dependence upon the cell body in the brain or cord is well demonstrated by the degeneration that occurs if severed. What then does the cell supply? Perhaps enzymes, for there is some evidence of an axonal migration of protein-like substances. The brain differs from the peripheral nerve in complexity, unit number, cell mixture, difficulty in dealing with single units and by having a greater susceptibility to its chemical environment. In the peripheral nerve there is a paucity of substrates whereas in the brain there is a superfluity. We are accustomed to think that the brain burns only glucose. This, however, is not true for the brain can and does burn other substances including glutamic acid.

It is quite apparent from these observations that considerable unit to unit, area to area, system to system differences occur in the resting brain and that further differences occur in the active state. That such differences exist is also borne out by the clinical symptomatology observed in different diseases. The polio virus exhibits an affinity for the enzyme systems of the motor nuclei which are also the choice of the agent in amyotrophic lateral sclerosis. Major seizures are precipitated by high CO_2 levels and petit mal seizures activated by low CO_2 values. In liver disease there are many symptoms reflecting different systems providing clinical support for a multifactor defect in hepatic encephalomyelopathy.

Up to this point this monograph has been concerned with clinical relationships. We must now give consideration to other possibilities of which there are many. The multiplicity of biochemical

TABLE XXXV

LIST OF KNOWN BIOCHEMICAL ABNORMALITIES IN HEPATIC DISEASE

Metabolite	Blood	Urine	Cerebro-spinal Fluid	Metabolite	Blood	Urine	Cerebro-spinal Fluid
Pyruvate	Increased	Increased	Increased	Vit A	Decreased	?	?
Amino acids	Increased	Increased		Vit B	Decreased	?	?
Bilirubin	Increased		Increased sometimes	Lactic acid	Increased	?	?
Bile Salts	Increased	?	?	Serum proteins	Decreased	?	?
Ammonia	Increased	?	?	Serum globulin	Increased	?	?
Poryphyrins	Increased	Increased	?	Blood ammonia	Increased	?	?
Hormones	Increased	?	?	Cholinesterase	Decreased	?	?
Antidiuretic hormone	Increased	?	?	Sugar, Galactose Fructose	Increased	?	?
Prothrombin	Decreased	?	?	Serum iron	Increased	?	?
Urobilinogen		Increased	?	Transaminase	Increased	?	?
Alkaline p'tase	Increased	?	?	Enzymes	?	?	?
Cholesterol	Increased	?	?	Leucopenia	Present	—	—
Cholesterol ester	Decreased	?	?	Anaemia	Present	—	—
Glycerol Fatty acids	Increased	?	?	Thrombocytopenia	Present	—	—
Phosphates	Increased	?	?	Others as yet unknown	?	—	—

alterations that reach the brain are listed in Table XXXV. Before the substances themselves can be discussed two important factors in brain metabolism need consideration—the blood—brain barrier and cerebral blood flow. These are factors which dictate to a great extent the responsivity and reactivity of the nervous system. Generally speaking the latter is a relatively stable organ whose metabolism rests largely on glucose and oxygen for the purposes of providing electrical energy by which means it operates. It is capable of manufacturing its own lipids and proteins and, of course, has its own enzyme systems. It is not, however, capable of manufacturing its own metals that aid the enzymes nor to manufacture its own carbohydrates except in unusual circumstances. It must rely upon building blocks supplied from the outside. Because of the nature of its function in controlling many bodily organs and systems, its metabolism is relatively stable, its blood vessels are different from those in other parts of the body and their control is under a different mechanism. In addition, the entire structure is protected by a rather formidable fortress—the blood-brain barrier. This barrier, like the wall of a fort allows a to and fro movement under normal conditions but may be breeched when circumstances are ripe. In any event when the brain is overcome, the route must be through the blood brain barrier.

The Blood Brain Barrier

All of the abnormal metabolites that result from hepatic disease soon come into contact with the blood brain barrier (BBB). Through this mechanism the brain becomes quite discriminative in admitting and rejecting substances to its domain. This is a device which is the recipient of considerable investigation today. While there are some seemingly nebulous aspects to this barrier it is known to consist of: (1) the capillary wall; (2) peri-capillary sheath; (3) pericapillary space; (4) neuroglial membrane; (5) the cerebral ground-substance composed chiefly of mucoprotein-mucocopolysaccaride complexes and quantities of hyaluronic acid; (6) perineuronal space, and (7) the neuronal cell membrane itself. The peri-neuronal space is a questionable entity whose form and existence is denied by the electron microscopists who believe this space as seen under light microscopy is a shrinkage or fixation artefact.

Considerable variation occurs in the amount, speed and size of particles than can penetrate this barrier. For example Na^{24}, Cl^{38} and K^{42} traverse the BBB at different rates, the latter being the slowest. H_2O, O_2 and anaesthetics pass the barrier so quickly as to render exact measurements impossible. Most substances, however, pass slower into the brain than into other organs. Large molecules and toxins do not pass at all, e.g., tetanus antitoxin, ceruloplasmin, penicillin. The velocity and intensity of passage varies with the location, it being greatest in the plexi, posterior hypophysis and the epiphysis. Passage through the BBB is also subject to topographical differences and in many instances the penetration is quicker in the cortex than in the white matter.

The white and gray matter behave differently to foreign fluids, e.g.: inflammatory exudates, fluid excesses. The neurones may show virtually no change in oedema due to hypoproteinemia because the O_2 diffusion is reduced only slightly. The white matter on the other hand may be severely demyelinated because of the high absorption of water by the myelin. Despite the integrity of neurones, the astrocytes may proliferate and under some conditions may undergo regressive changes and be transformed into "naked nuclei" (Alzheimer cells) as in hepatolenticular degeneration (325). Thus, we have in these observations possible explanation for the cerebral alteration both pathological and symptomatic for they may be related to fluid changes irrespective of any other biochemical defects.

Numerous substances can cause a breakdown of the blood brain barrier. Those which are pertinent to liver disease are as follows:

(1) Bile Salts—Na glycocholate (0.5%) concentration (313-315).
　　　　　　　—Na desoxycholate (0.4%) concentration.
(2) Bilirubin (316).
(3) Large quantities of physiological agents (313).
(4) C^{14}, Cu^{64}, K^{42}, Na^{24}, S^{35}, Zn^{65}, P^{32} (317).
(5) Methionine S^{35} (318).

The BBB is not affected by vasodilation, histamine or acetylcholine and it is not altered by physiological means.

This is but a partial list and further study will advance our knowledge of its selectivity. It is apparent that great consideration must be given to the BBB in this relationship. It is quite possible that preliminary breakdown of the BBB by such as bile salts or bilirubin may spearhead the way for further biochemical changes.

Cerebral Blood Flow

As a result of innumerable studies Kety (319) has pegged the normal cerebral blood flow (CBF) at 54 cubic centimeters per 100 grams of brain tissue per minute. The normal oxygen consumption is 3.3 cubic centimeters in the same amount of tissue.

In diabetic coma he has found an increase in the CBF to 65 cc/100 gm./min. and a similar increase in insulin coma to 63 cc./100 gm./min. Since there are about 2 grams of glycogen in the whole human brain which are readily convertible to glucose, the brain is able to withstand the effects of hypoglycemia much better than anoxia. It can be calculated that the glycogen of the brain will support cerebral metabolism for about 90 minutes at the low level present in coma. After the glycogen supplies are depleted the enzyme systems turn cannibalistic and commence to devour the structural components of the neurone! The situation in hepatic coma appears to be different.

Wechsler, Crum and Roth (232) studied the cerebral blood flow and O_2 consumption in seven cases of hepatic coma. In each there was an alkalosis (to be discussed later) with an average pH of about 7.48. There was no change in the cerebral vascular resistance (CVR) but the arterial pCO_2 was depressed to 25 mm. Hg. Despite the constant CVR the CBF fell significantly to 33 cc./100 gm./min. partly as a result of a drop in the mean arterial blood pressure (MABP) to 78 mm. Hg. The decrease in the CBF and the lack of change in the arterio-venous O_2 difference (AVO₂) indicated a low cerebral metabolic rate (CMRO₂) of about 1.7 cc./100 gm./min. or about half of the normal rate. Since there is a normal arterial oxygen concentration in the blood reaching the brain the reason for the low cerebral metabolic rate is due to deficiencies in the enzyme systems that enable the brain to use oxygen.

Similar studies were recently reported by Fazekas, Ticktin, Ehrmantraut and Alman (320). In this report the patients were divided into three groups of hepatic insufficiency, *viz.*, those without cerebral manifestations, those with lethargy, somnolence and confusion and a third group with coma. A summary of the article by Fazekas is shown in Table XXXVI. It is apparent from this that the chief difference in the groups reported is that of a reduced cerebral oxygen utilization to a level about one half of the normal. The depression of oxygen utilization cannot be entirely the result of increased blood ammonia levels or an increased uptake since the values of ammonia were not significantly different

TABLE XXXVI

CEREBRAL METABOLISM IN HEPATIC INSUFFICIENCY

| | Group Average Values | | | |
	Group I 20 Patients	Group II 15 Patients	Group III 16 Patients	Normal Values
Age	52	53	54	
CBF	47.1	41.9	39.6	54
CMRO$_2$	2.3	1.7	1.6	3.3
CVR	2.0	2.0	1.7	
MABP	90	77	65	
AVO$_2$	5.14	4.41	4.07	6.6
Art. NH$_3$	1.7	1.9	2.6	
Vein NH$_3$	1.5	1.7	2.4	
Art. pyruvic	1.8	2.4	2.5	
Vein pyruvic	1.7	2.3	2.2	

(Modified from Fazekas *et al.* (332)).

in groups 1 and 2. Furthermore the authors reported that 10 normal individuals exhibited the same ammonia differences and a similar ammonia uptake as was noted in the cases of hepatic insufficiency. They could find no good correlation between blood ammonia levels and neurological manifestations.

The diminished CMRO$_2$ indicates a disturbance in carbohydrate metabolism but this is not due to low blood sugar values since the latter are usually within normal limits. The value must be due to improper utilization of oxygen, a fact which is supported by the high blood pyruvate levels suggesting a defect in pyruvic oxidase systems. The energy derived from such reactions is required in reductive amination of glutamic acid and if reduced may as a result cause impairment of keto-acid oxidation which in turn may be responsible for the elevated blood ammonia levels as well as the accumulation of pyruvate. The practical therapeutic application of this lies in the intravenous administration of vitamin B compounds or other respiratory enzyme precursors. Oxygen itself is not needed since the arterial oxygen saturation is normal. The utilization, however, is imperfect.

The control of the cerebral blood vessels is largely under the influence of CO$_2$. The role played by the alkalosis in hepatic coma is discussed below. These observations further suggest the possibility that the cerebral alterations could be due to a relative anoxia. The pathological cell changes certainly would mirror this alteration. Although it is unlikely that the myelin or astrocytic changes would. Such observations further strengthen the multiple factor hypothesis.

Alkalosis and Electrolyte Imbalances

Disturbances in body electrolytes and fluids are known to occur in hepatic diseases. Eisenmenger, Blondheim, Bongiovanni and Kunkel (321), Kunkel (322), Chalmers (323) and Mark (324) demonstrated the retention of sodium in patients with ascites. This is due to the stimulus of a constant state of dehydration and correlates with a low serum sodium. As a result of this, one would expect a shift in the sodium-potassium balance. Ascites is not due entirely to hypoalbuminuria, or portal hypertension since antidiuretic substances have been found in cirrhotics by Iverson (325), Chalmers (323), and Mark (324). Chalmers studied the fluid balances in cirrhosis and noted hemoconcentration and dehydration during the development of ascites and shifts in sodium and potassium. The latter has been recently noted to exert considerable influence upon nervous system function. The retention of fluids in cirrhosis provokes the question of cerebral oedema as a cause of the cerebral symptoms.

Few studies have been made on these abnormalities in hepatic coma. Amatuzio, Stutzman, Shrifter and Nesbitt (326) studied this aspect of hepatic coma and noted a decrease in sodium, chlorides and plasma CO_2 values. Vanamee, Poppell, Glicksman, Randall and Roberts (327) studied 29 patients with hepatic coma, 25 of which had respiratory alkalosis as manifest by high pH and low pCO_2 values. There was also a coincident elevation of blood ammonia levels. No correlation was observed between the latter and the symptomatology of hepatic decompensation. The elevated ammonia levels, however, may stimulate respiratory exchange and aid in the development of the alkalosis. The characteristics of the oxyhemoglobin dissociation curve under conditions of high pH and low CO_2 indicates impaired O_2 unloading at the tissue levels (328). In respiratory alkalosis the electrographic changes are similar to those reported in ammonia toxicity according to Darrow and Pathman (329). It was further noted that the hypocapnia causes destruction of acetylcholine by cholinesterase. The control of CO_2 over the cerebral blood vessels has been mentioned and one can surmise an additive effect of the low CO_2 preventing any compensatory vasodilation that might be needed as a result of other metabolic abnormalities and thereby contribute to the coma. It is apparent from such observations that electrolyte and fluid alterations resulting from impaired liver function cannot be ignored as important factors in the production of coma. Further studies are needed on this aspect.

Enzymes and Metalloenzymes

Enzyme research has done much in the past decade to explain the role of organic micronutrients such as thiamine, riboflavin, nicotinamide, pyridoxine and others. Progress has been made also in establishing and clarifying the role of bulk metals as K, Na, Ca, Mg, and Fe as well as that of the trace metals, Cu, CO, Mn, Zn, Mo, Ni, Ba, As and Al. Physiological control over the metallo-enzyme activity is affected by the availability of the ion plus the effect of trace metal antagonists. Thus, many of these enzyme systems work under extremely close tolerances and their functions are readily prevented by abnormal amounts, whether excess of deficiencies, of metals.

There are approximately 25 different enzyme systems in the brain and perhaps more, a knowledge of which is imperfect and many of which are also present in other organs as well, such as the ubiquitous catalase. Cytochrome C is closely linked with iron and is discussed under Iron Metabolism. The relationship of these to the basal ganglia and porphyrin metabolism are also discussed in the paragraph on Porphyrin Metabolism.

The phosphatase enzymes of the brain have been studied by Feigin and Wolf (330). In general the phosphatases catalyze the liberation of inorganic PO_4 from phosphate esters. Several of these exist. Alkaline phosphatase splits a variety of phosphate mono-esters such as glycerophosphate, glucose-1-phosphate, creatine phosphate, hexosephosphate, and nucleotides as adenylic acid and ATP. It is activated by magnesium and inhibited by cyanides. Acid phosphatase, 5-nucleotidase, phosphoamidase, pyrophosphatases and adenosine triphosphatase are other important enzymes whose normal function is understood but whose functions have not been studied in this relationship.

Roizin (331) has studied the oxidases in various diseases of the brain. The oxidases are capable of catalyzing reactions of oxidation. Cytochrome oxidase, phenolase, purinoxidases, succinoxidases, tyrosinase are members of this group. Some of these are inhibited by the action of bile salts. Ceruloplasmin, the copper containing globulin compound has the oxidase activity and other members of this group are also copper containing substances. They are generally inhibited by sulfides, cyanides and metal binding ions and by deficiencies of copper.

Vitamin B compounds are enzymes essential for carbohydrate metabolism and are discussed briefly under the paragraph on carbohydrate metabolism.

Metals play an important part in enzyme systems. Cu, Fe and Zn are discussed separately. Magnesium is the important ion in decarboxylation enzymes which catalyze carboxylase, pyruvic acid oxidase and alpha-keto gutaric oxidase. This ion is also important in the action of phophatases, hexokinase, arginine—ATP transphosphorylase, enolase, alkaline and acid phosphatases. Zinc is important in alkaline phosphatase and carbonic anhydrase systems. The latter is essential to the elimination of CO_2 and is therefore important in respiratory gas exchange.

Only a few isolated facts concerning these enzyme systems are available now since they have not been studied with reference to hepatic-cerebral relationships. A study of these is highly desirable.

Copper Metabolism

The recent observation of an increase in the urinary excretion of copper in hepatolenticular degeneration has focused attention of the metabolism of this substance. Copper is transported in the blood in two fractions: (a) ceruloplasmin—an indirect re-acting fraction, and (b) a direct re-acting fraction.

Ceruloplasmin, a copper containing protein was first isolated by Holmberg and Laurell (332, 333) in 1947. It is an alpha-globulin with a molecular weight of 150,000, and contains 0.34 per cent copper and has the enzymatic activity of an oxidase. Ninety-five per cent of the blood copper exists in this form. Ceruloplasmin is not found in the brain but is present in small quantities in the liver and kidney according to Markowitz, Gubler, Mahoney, Cartwright and Wintrobe (262).

The direct reacting or "loose" copper fraction constitutes about 5 per cent of serum copper and it is bound to the albumin fraction. Together, these two forms make up the total plasma copper the normal value of which is about 116 micrograms per 100 cubic centimeters of plasma. Although the bulk of the plasma copper is in the form of ceruloplasmin, this element is transported in the direct reacting or albumin fraction. Oral or intravenous administered radiocopper, Cu^{64}, appears first in the albumin fraction and later in the globulin fraction or ceruloplasmin according to Gubler (334). The copper content of the red blood cells is 115 micrograms per 100 cubic centimeters of packed red blood cells.

Copper has a widespread distribution and the average adult ingestion is 2.5 milligrams of Cu per day so that man maintains a balance of about 2 milligrams per day. Because of its ubiquity it is doubtful if copper deficincy can occur in man except in marked hypoproteinemia for it cannot be entirely excluded from the diet.

Copper is stored in the liver and other organs with a greater amount in the latter because of the relatively greater mass although the liver is the chief storage point. Copper is also found in the brain (324). Copper is excreted in the bile and this amount varies between 0 to 70 micrograms per day regardless of the route of administration. According to van Ravestyn (335) some bile is excreted through the intestinal wall and of a given oral dose of copper, 65 to 75 per cent is recovered in the feces and only 25 per cent absorbed into the body. A rise in serum copper occurs after the intravenous administration of copper and in a few days there is a rise in the biliary and fecal copper levels. Seventy-two per cent of radiocopper (Cu^{64}) is recovered in the stools and 1 per cent in the urine according to Bush, Mahoney, Markowitz, Gubler,

Cartwright, and Wintrobe (270). The normal urinary copper excretion is 0 to 25 micrograms per 24 hours.

There are several copper containing proteins and enzymes in mammalian tissues: (1) Butyl co-enzyme, a dehydrogenase which catalyzes the first step in the oxidation of 3-8 carbon atom fatty acids. (2) *Uricase,* links copper to purine metabolism. (3) *Tyrosinase,* another copper containing enzyme that links copper to melanin metabolism by catalyzing the oxidation of L-tyrosine to L-dihydroxy-phenylalanine (DOPA) and to melanin pigments. (4) Hepatocuprein, hemocuprein and the milk copper proteins have not been functionally categorized at present. (5) Ceruloplasmin exhibits a nonspecific oxidase activity. Copper is necessary for the activity of the cytochrome oxidase complex and these place copper in a fundamental position in oxidation-reduction and energy transfer reactions.

In the lower animals, copper is necessary for the production of wool and the maintenance of the myelin sheath. It is antagonistic to zinc and molybdenum and a high concentration of zinc will result in a copper deficiency (334).

Copper deficiency occurs in animals, the best known example of which is the Enzootic ataxia of sheep. It was first described by Bennetts and Chapman (336) who studied this condition in the lambs in Australia, and by Dunlop, Innes, Shearer and Wells (337) who studied a similar condition in England. At autopsy these animals exhibited demyelination of the spinal cord, particularly of the dorsal spinocerebellar tracts, increased deposition of hemosiderin in the liver and a low serum copper (336-338). The addition of copper to the feed of pregnant ewes prevented this condition from developing in the lambs. Gross cavitation of the brain occurs in acute copper poisoning according to these authors. In these animals the tissue copper is very high and when a sudden egress of copper from tissues occur, the kidneys are damaged and the animal dies. If the animal survives these crises he develops a cirrhosis. The hypocupremia of these animals is accompanied by hypoferremia, bone marrow hyperplasia, retarded bone growth and anaemia. A deficiency of copper does not occur in man as a result of dietary means. Hypocupremia in man occurs in hepatolenticular degeneration, the sprue and the nephrotic syndrome. Campbell, Daniel, Porter, Russell, Smith and Innes (339) reported on the development of neurological symptoms indistinguishable from multiple sclerosis amongst laboratory technicians working on the copper deficient lambs in England. No abnormalities of copper could be found in these individuals, however.

Cumings (54) analyzed the copper content of 27 normal brains and found the highest values in the globus pallidus, and putamen. These areas had also the highest iron values. He established a normal range of 1.2 to 8.2 milligrams of copper per 100 grams of white matter and a value of 1.2 to 7.2 milligrams per 100 grams of grey matter. Tingey (340) demonstrated a progressive increase in the copper content of the brain with the development of the nervous system. The brain of the newborn infant is low in copper but reaches the adult level at approximately 2 years of age. Mandelbrot and associates (259) concluded that while copper is essential for the development of the fiber tracts, function is not disturbed by an excess or deficiency of copper after the developmental period is past. The low copper content of the infant nervous system and its progressive increase suggests a relationship to myelinization of the nervous system. A further link between copper and myelin metabolism is to be found in the work of Klüver (341) who noted a progressive porphyrization of the nervous system which was believed to parallel the formation of myelin. Porphyrin metabolism is intimately related to copper metabolism.

The exact action of copper is obscure. Its presence in many organs indicates a definite function. It has been considered as a catalyst for the formation of hemoglobin by Dry (245), for the oxidation of cysteine and glutathione by Elvehjem (342), for the breakdown of glycogen by Kiel and Nelson (343) and for the formation of melanin by Flesch (344). According to Kiel and Nelson, copper is necessary for erythropoiesis, pigmentation and myelination and it plays an important role in the function of cytochrome, catalase, and oxidase systems which are necessary for cellular respiration. Glazebrook (53) regarded copper as an enzyme inhibitor, similar to other heavy metals. The basal ganglia are invested with a very rich vascular system which is indicative of a high oxygen demand and this area is susceptible to carbon monoxide and cyanides which are known enzyme inhibitors. According to Glazebrook (53) the concentration of copper in the basal ganglia in Wilson's disease may be 50 times the normal, and certainly sufficient to cause inhibition of enzymes and ultimately necrosis.

While the precise role of copper in cerebrohepatic disease remains hidden in a maze of chemical reactions it would appear to play some role in the production of cerebral symptomatology. There is no assurance, however, that copper in itself is the cause of cerebral changes nor is it possible to determine whether the defect in copper metabolism is the primary one or merely the side effect of some more basic disturbance. Cerebral symptoms not infrequently arise from defective carbohyrate and porphyrin metabolism, both of which are in a large measure dependent upon the metabolism of copper.

At present it can only be stated that some disturbance of copper exists in certain hepatic diseases and that neurological disturbances have been noted in conditions with defective copper metabolism.

Iron Metabolism

Hemochromatosis, infectious hepatitis, and portal cirrhosis have been known to be associated with an elevated serum iron (345-358). The cerebral changes in these conditions have been mentioned and the question is now raised as to the role of iron in the development of these alterations.

Iron is necessary for the functions of hematopoiesis (359), and cellular respiration, both of which if seriously disturbed are capable of altering cerebral function.

In the blood, iron is attached to the hemoglobin molecule and in the serum to the globulin fraction of the serum proteins (360). Since it has already been observed that an iron deficiency anaemia occurs in a large percentage of hepatic diseases a paradoxical situation with respect to iron exists. On the one hand there is an iron deficiency anemia manifest by a reduction of iron in the red blood cells and on the other hand, there is an increase in the serum iron. While distinctly abnormal the exact significance of this is not clear and the question of an autointoxication with iron has been raised. An elevated serum iron may effect cerebral metabolism in several ways. First by an indirect effect upon copper with which iron seems to have a reciprocal relationship (342). Both elements are necessary for hematopoiesis and cellular respiration and cannot be functionally separated. Secondly, an abnormality of iron may directly affect cellular respiration.

The brain is dependent upon oxygen for its existence and iron plays a very important part in the utilization of this substance. The mechanism of cellular respiration has been extensively studied by Warburg and Christian (360-363), Keilin and Hartree (364, 365), Himwich (366), Embden, Denticke, and Kraft (367), Meyerhof (368), Cori (369) and found to be controlled by iron, peroxidase, catalase and cytochromes. Of these, iron and cytochrome are the most important in so far as cerebral cellular respiration is concerned. Not only is oxygen conveyed to the brain by the iron in hemoglobin but upon its arrival its transfer is mediated from hemoglobin to the cell by the action of iron. This transfer of oxygen is due to the capacity of elemental iron to take up oxygen whereupon the molecule becomes trivalent and upon surrendering oxygen it is reduced to a bivalent substance. During this process oxygen is transferred to the cell. While this seems simple enough it is much more complex and involves cytochrome, a cellular respiratory enzyme and which is basically a porphyrin compound with one atom of iron (370-372). It may be said here in passing that iron is present in every cell and serves not only in the transfer of oxygen but it also binds the corresponding chromagen which is characterized by a prophyrin structure. The chromagen of bone marrow is hemoglobin, that of the muscle is myoglobin and of other tissues is cytochrome. Cytochrome is an iron containing enzyme which catalyzes the transfer of oxygen to a utilizable form.

Because cerebral respiration is dependent upon oxygen it is not surprising to find substantial quantities of iron in the brain. The high concentration of iron and copper in the globus pallidus and putamen has been mentioned. Spatz (373) and Ferroni (374) found the greatest concentration of iron in the substantia nigra and globus pallidus. Lesser quantities are present in the dentate nucleus, red nucleus and subthalamic body of Luys, while the cortex, amygdaloid nucleus and mammillary bodies contain the least amounts. This distribution of iron is interesting and parallels the distribution of cytochromes which were demonstrated in the same areas and in the same relative amounts by Klüver (341).

Hyperferremia may cause cerebral symptoms and after the introduction of Blaud's pills in 1832 iron poisoning was common. In recent years more cases of iron intoxication have been noted following the use of inorganic iron salts. Napier (375), in 1936, reported a case in which the patient received 468 grains of ferrous sulphate and developed status epilepticus. Birch and Hill (376), in 1951, reported a case of anaemia for which saccharated ferric oxide containing 100 milligrams of iron in 10 cubic centimeters of vehicle was given intravenously after which the patient developed headache, nausea, became drowsy, stuporous, developed focal seizures and elapsed into coma.

Peterson (377), in 1952, noted an elevated serum iron in 92 per cent of his cases of acute hepatitis. This was considered an unexpected finding in view of the fact that the serum iron is depressed in most infections. Peterson postulated several theories to account for this; namely, increased absorption of iron from the gastrointestinal tract; decreased utilization of iron for hemoglobin formation; decreased excretion of iron in the bile and blocked iron deposition in the liver due to inflammation. Kipping and Schmoldt (378) noted that the serum iron was at its maximum concentration during the acute stages of hepatitis but could find no correlation with other liver function tests.

The relationship of hemochromatosis to Wilson's Disease has been mentioned. McDougal and Adams (52) studied 29 cases of hemochromatosis, 10 of which died in hepatic coma. They concluded that the brain was affected in this disease directly by the deposition of pigment and indirectly by alterations of the parenchyma and supporting tissues. Two pigments are found in the liver and brain in hemochromatosis (379-381). Hemosiderin, an organic compound of iron, is the most abundant. Hemofuchsin.

iron free, identical with the pigment of atrophy and old age and found in large quantities in the skin is a melanin precursor for whose metabolism copper is necessary. This is present in hemochromatotic livers in smaller quantities. Both are found in the brain. Bronzing due to hemofuchsin has been noted in the area postrema (382) and choroid plexus of the fourth ventricle. Hemosiderin has been found in the area postrema, pituitary stalk, hypothalamus, corpus Luysi, dentate nucleus and choroid plexus of lateral and third ventricles (380) in hemochromatosis. A pronounced hyperplasia of astrocytes was noted by McDougal and Adams (52) who related glial and neuronal changes to hepatic failure.

Although hyperferremia exists in some hepatic diseases and in itself is known to cause cerebral symptoms, it is not the sole cause of cerebral alterations for the serum iron is normal in obstructive cirrhosis.

It is impossible to determine whether this abnormality of iron metabolism is a primary disorder or a defect secondary to some other basic disturbance. Pyridoxine deficiency is swine is accompanied by an enormous deposition of iron in the liver (383). Cartwright (359) noted that a deficiency of cobalt cause a marked increase in the deposition of iron in the tissues and Herbut, Watson and Perkins (384) noted a similar effect in the experimental production of diabetes with alloxan. It is apparent that iron plays an important part in cerebral function and disturbances in iron exist in many hepatic diseases. However, like copper, the exact role is obscure and further studies are indicated.

Amino Acid Metabolism

The occurrence of aminoacidemia in hepatic insufficiency was first noted in 1914 by Chesney, Marshall and Rowntree (89). Six years later Stadie and van Slyke (90) observed an increase in titratable amino acids in hepatic coma and concluded that these acids were formed by the autolysis of degenerating liver and an inability to deaminate amino acids. Mann (385), in 1927, arrived at the same conclusion as a result of hepatic artery ligation in Eck fistulized dogs. It has been previously shown by van Slyke and

Meyer (386) that orally administered amino acids were quickly transformed into ammonia and the importance of the liver as a deaminator was demonstrated by Bollman, Mann and Magath (387) who demonstrated the inability of hepatectomized dogs to deaminate amino acids. It was also shown that approximately 80 per cent of the liver must be extirpated or destroyed before symptoms of hepatic insufficiency appear. The amino-acid nitrogen concentration of the plasma is 3 to 6 milligrams per 100 cubic centimeters and constitutes the equilibrium of amino acids absorbed from the intestines and supplemented by tissue protein fractions. The liver is the chief site of de-amination, transamination and amidation a function which remains unaltered until about 90 per cent of the liver is functionally destroyed. After absorption, the amino acids serve as precursors or constituents of vitamins, hormones, co-enzymes, detoxication products, tissue proteins and enzyme systems.

The excretion of amino acids usually parallels the plasma levels except in Wilson's disease and in the de Toni-Fanconi syndrome. Most of the amino acids in the glomerular filtrate are reabsorbed in the tubules but are not all reabsorbed to the same degree. The essential amino acids are retained preferentially. Some amino acids compete with each other for tubular reabsorption as evidenced by the loading of an individual with lysine which interferes with the reabsorption of arginine. Amino aciduria can result from high blood levels and may occur in hepatic necrosis, muscular atrophies, hyperthyroidism, burns and carcinomatosis. It can also arise from renal tubular failure as a result of nephrosis, allergic states, lupus, pituitary disease and the de Toni-Fanconi syndrome and lastly it can occur without renal lesions and in face of normal blood levels as occurs in hepatolenticular degeneration and cystinuria.

Proteins, purines, pyramidines, choline, sphingosine as well as amino acids constitute a pool from which the building blocks of protein synthesis are drawn and to which they are returned during the disintegration of proteins. This provides a relatively constant supply of such substances. In severe hepatic disease the liver is unable to cope with its function of deamination and amino acids accumulate and may spill into the urine. Dent and Walshe (92), in 1951, showed abnormalities in more than one amino acid in mild liver injury and that the amount of aminoaciduria increased with the severity of the liver damage. In acute hepatic failure all amino acids were excreted in excess and in chronic hepatic diseases cystine, beta-aminoisobutyric acid, and histidine were increased.

In hepatic coma, Walshe (61), Blass, Cochin and Durlach (388), Schreier (389), and Dent and Walshe (92) have noted gross aminoaciduria. Similarly in hepatolenticular degeneration, Uzman and Brown (91), Porter (248), Cooper, Eckhardt, Faloon and Davidson (94), and Deverdier (93) observed elevations of amino acids in the blood and urine. In most of these cases the hepatic disease was fairly far advanced. On the other hand Roman (95), Greene (390), and Murphy, Chalmers, Eckhardt and Davidson (144) could find no elevation of amino acids in their cases of hepatic coma.

Walshe (61) investigated 18 cases of hepatic coma and noted an abnormal pattern of amino acid excretion in all cases despite normal blood levels. He concluded that the neurological involvement was due to a breakdown in the mechanism of regulation and liberation of potentially toxic amounts of certain amino acids. It has been shown that some amino acids are more toxic than others. An excess of cystine was shown by Earle and Victor (391), in 1942, to result in hemorrhagic necrosis of the liver. Morehead, Fishman and Artom (392) found tubular necrosis of the kidney from excess of serine. The intravenous administration of protein hydrolysates have been known to cause convulsions, vomiting and pain. Glycine and alanine were shown by Mann (385), in 1927, to be toxic to Eck fistulized dogs but not to normal animals. Diets deficient in sulfur amino acids and tocopherols will cause hepatic necrosis which is accompanied by a rise in the blood glutathione and in aminoaciduria.

Glutamic acid is a more important amino acid in cerebral metabolism than the others and indeed the concentration of this substance in the brain is higher than in any other organ (299, 393, 394). This is characteristic of the unmyelinated as well as the myelinated brain and it remains constant during the period of myelination. Quastel and Wheatley (299), Krebs (395) demonstrated the slow metabolism of glutamic acid by the brain with the liberation of glutamine and ammonia. Mayer, Gross and Walker (396) were able to restore to consciousness 26 of 45 patients in hypoglycemic coma by the intravenous administration of glutamic acid. Weil and Malherbe (97) demonstrated that glutamic acid takes part in amination, transamination and amidation all three of which bind ammonia and not only remove it from the nervous system but also provide a source of ammonia for other reactions.

Glutamic acid and glutamine may both enter the brain or one may enter and the other be produced as a result of enzyme action or the nucleus of one may be formed through the tricarboxylic cycle. There is evidence both for an extracerebral source and also that it may be formed from ammonia and ketoglutaric acid (312). Experimental studies indicate that the brain fails to take up this amino acid from the circulating blood as the blood brain barrier appears to block the uptake of glutamic acid by the brain. These observations would indicate that any benefit from glutamic acid thereby would not be the result of direct cerebral effect but rather a peripheral action. The failure of this substance to alter the course of hepatic coma in some cases further supports the contention that elevations of blood ammonia are not the only cause of the comatose state. Walshe (197) reported an excess of glutamine in the sera of 3 of 18 patients in hepatic coma. Methiomine sulfoxide which inhibits this action of glutamic acid according to Borek, Miller, Sheiness and Waelsch (397), and Waelsch, Owades, Miller and Borek (398), was noted in the spinal fluid of 2 patients reported by Walshe (197). Schreier (389) examined the sera of 23 patients with varied liver disease and demonstrated an increase of methionine in all cases in which the hepatic disease was severe. The urinary excretion of this substance was normal except in 5 cases of cirrhosis in which it was elevated.

Excesses of other individual amino acids have been determined by chromatography (92). Tyrosine and phenylalanine were found in the urine of cirrhotics in 90 and 60 per cent of the cases, respectively, by Blass, Cochin and Durlach (388). In the same cases alanine and glutamine were elevated in the sera.

Glutamic acid is converted to alpha keto-glutaric acid by oxidation and deamination. The latter is readily converted to pyruvic acid. Walshe feels that in the event of an interference in the equation

Glutamic acid $\rightleftharpoons$ alpha keto-glutaric acid $\rightleftharpoons$ pyruvic acid

by virtue of a reduced availability of alpha keto-glutaric acid ATP (adenosine triphosphate) is needed to carry out this equation and this results in a disruption of the carbohydrate cycle. Glutamine was elevated in the spinal fluid in all cases of hepatic coma reported by Walshe.

In the light of our present knowledge of amino acid metabolism it is difficult to assess the role of individual amino acids. Many of the amino acids are elevated in hepatic diseases of all varieties. Emphasis seems to be placed on the glutamic acid and upon methionine in so far as the cerebral changes are concerned at this time. The exact action of excess acids on the brain is not known and several possibilities have been mentioned among which are: (1) that glutamic acid in excess disturbs the normal equilibrium with ammonia so that the latter accumulates; (2) that methionine inhibits the activity of glutamine and prevents it from removing ammonia; (3) that glutamine in excess disrupts the carbohydrate cycle and that neurological manifestations are due to the latter phenomena.

It will be noted later that the amino acids are constituents of the cytochromes, A, B and C and the disruption of the function of this substance by excesses or deficiencies of amino acids is a possibility that has not been explored.

Carbohydrate Metabolism

Hypoglycaemia, once postulated as the cause of cerebral manifestations in hepatic disease does not occur. Low blood sugar values were not found in any of the 82 cases presented in this thesis nor in the cases reported by Walshe (81), and Murphy, Chalmers, Eckhardt and Davidson (144). The coma of hepatic insufficiency does not respond to glucose infusions and in this respect it differs from that of the hepatectomized dog which exhibits a remarkable response to parenteral glucose. Hyperglycaemia may be found in any series of hepatic diseases and especially if hemochromatosis is included, but the neurological symptoms are not due to this alone.

Despite this, however, abnormalities of carbohydrate metabolism are known to occur in hepatic disease. Such defects are not due to the excess or deficiency of glucose per se but rather, are due to the improper utilization and breakdown of carbohydrate in the brain. This may be affected by a variety of factors, some of which have been discussed; *viz.*, defects in copper, iron and amino acid metabolism. In addition, the metabolism of glucose is dependent upon enzymes many of which are vitamins, in the manufacture of which, the liver is concerned.

Bondy (399) has listed the following defects in carbohydrate metabolism in hepatic disease.

(1) Inadequate maintenance of blood glucose.
(2) Slow clearance of exogenous glucose.
(3) Mild diabetic-type glucose curve.
(4) Ribose deficiency.

From a study of tissue slices Warburg (361, 362) demonstrated the high degree of anaerobic glycosis that occurs in the brain. In this process, lactic acid is formed, the energy for which is derived from the high energy phosphate bonds of ATP (adenosine triphosphate). In addition, three enzyme systems, the coenzyme, adenylic and cocarboxylase, are necessary for the metabolism of glucose (400). All three contain vitamin substances, nicotinamide, adenylic acid, and thiamine. All tissues, especially the liver, store diphosphothiamine where it can be dephosphorylated and free thiamine supplied to the blood.

Williams and Bissell (401) demonstrated and impaired cocarboxylase formation from thiamine in liver disease. Snell and Butt (99) noted an elevation of the lactic acid and pyruvic acid levels of the blood in hepatic coma and observed a response to the administration of glucose, niacin and thiamine. They postulated that hepatic coma was the result of an abnormal carbohydrate utilization related to deficiencies in vitamin B.

Diphosphothiamine was shown by Peters (402), in 1936, to be necessary for the oxidation of pyruvate in the brain and in thiamine-deficient states the amount of diphosphothiamine in the tissues is markedly decreased. Amatuzio and Nesbitt (98) investigated pyruvate metabolism and found it elevated in hepatic coma. They believed the liver failed to take up pyruvic acid to form the dicarboxylic acids necessary for the Kreb's cycle and hence a defect in aerobic carbohydrate metabolism existed in hepatic disease.

The effect of the blood constituents upon the uptake of glucose was studied by Geiger, Magnes, Taylor, and Veralli (403). By perfusion of an isolated brain with blood which had been previously passed through an isolated liver it was shown that the uptake of glucose from the blood fluctuated, despite a constant O_2 concentration and cerebral blood flow. It was further shown that in deep narcosis or after anoxia the glucose uptake became steady and constant. From this it seemed apparent that the transfer of glucose was interrupted but was restored promptly by the addition of fresh liver extract. Improvement of a lesser degree was obtained by the addition of whole blood. Aside from the application here to glucose it is quite possible that a similar relationship exists which governs the uptake of other substances by the brain. We must not assume that each substance is independent and taken up by the brain irrespective and independent of other substances.

Although a great many facts are known about cerebral and hepatic carbohydrate metabolisms so many details are lacking that it is impossible to evaluate the role of carbohydrates in the production of cerebral symptoms at this time. One can only speculate that some defect exists probably within the enzymatic system which provides a utilizable form of fuel for cellular consumption.

Prophyrin Metabolism

The excretion of urinary coproporphyrin has been mentioned as a sensitive index of hepatic function. Watson, Sutherland and Hawkinson (121) studied coproporphyrin excretion in cirrhosis and found it elevated in 94 per cent of the cases. While no definite correlation was found between the extent of the cirrhosis and the clinical features of the disease, in general the more moribund the patient the greater the excretion of coproporphyrin. In all instances where mental disturbances were observed the urinary coproporphyrin excretion was elevated. Similar elevations of coproporphyrin excretion were found in infectious hepatitis and obstructive jaundice. In the former instance the type I isomer was increased whereas in the latter, the type III isomer was elevated. Nesbitt (187) studied the daily urinary coproporphyrin excretion in 4 patients in acute hepatic insufficiency with episodic neurologic symptoms ranging from mild disorientation to frank psychoses and coma. Prior to and during each episode of acute insufficiency the excretion of coproporphyrin decreased only to rise again when neurological symptoms disappeared.

Acquired porphyria has long been known to have neurological manifestations evident clinically and pathologically. Baker and Watson (404) reported on the pathological changes in acute porphyria which in general were quite similar to those observed in hepatic disease. Porphyrin compounds are readily identified by a characteristic fluorescence and absorption spectrum. Study of the brain of a recent case of acute porphyria which remained in coma for 10 days showed the presence of porphyrins in the sixth nerve, optic nerve, hypothalamus, and scattered areas of cortex, cerebellum and brain stem and demyelination was noted in the sixth nerve. It is evident from this that some forms of porphyrin are "toxic" to the nervous system. This may be due to the inhibitory effect of porphyrins on cellular respiration.

On the other hand Klüver (341) has shown the presence of naturally occurring porphyrins in the central nervous system. He found the emission spectrum of porphyrins in the white matter, optic, fifth, seventh and eighth cranial nerves. Porphyrin compounds were not found in the third, fourth and sixth cranial nerves, basal ganglia or cortex.

Klüver (341) also found that the porphyrin content of the brain parallels the myelin and he stated that the progressive myelination of the developing nervous system is accompanied by a progressive ascending porphyrinization. The exact location and function of porphyrins in the formation and metabolism of lipids is unknown but there is good evidence for the existence of some relationship.

The porphyrin ring is the basic structure of most of the body chromogens including hemoglobin, myoglobin, bilirubin, and cytochrome (372). The latter is a respiratory enzyme present in the brain and liver and closely related to porphyrins. The arrangement of the side chains on the porphyrin nucleus of cytochrome is identical with protoporphyrin and hemoglobin. Cytochrome in addition to having a basic porphyrin structure is composed of 16 different amino acids, 6 atoms of sulfur and one of iron. In the general scheme of cellular respiration the action of cytochrome C is due in part to the presence of iron but primarily it is considered as an electron carrier. Nerve cells are rich in cytochrome C but none is found in the white matter. The parallel distribution of iron and cytochrome in the brain has been mentioned. The absence of cytochrome in areas where porphyrins are present has been observed, by Klüver (341) and is worthy of note. The substantia nigra and cerebral cortex are particularly rich in cytochrome C. The cytochrome oxidase system catalyzes the greatest part of the oxygen utilized in cerebral metabolism and in the absence of cytochrome of its oxidase, cellular oxidation is at a minimum. Cytochrome does not appear in the embryo (405) which is in line with the low cerebral oxygen uptake at this time of development.

In hepatectomized rats the cytochrome is low and regenerating hepatic cells are accompanied by a rise in liver cytochrome (372, 406). The toxic effect of cyanides and carbon monoxide on cerebral functions is due primarily to the inhibitory action of these substances on the activity of cytocrome and this has been amply illustrated by Warburg (407) who noted that the absorption spectrum of ferricytochrome was completely abolished by cyanide and carbon monoxide.

Porphyrin synthesis is related to copper metabolism and Lemberg and Legge (372) have noted an acceleration of porphyrin synthesis in the presence of copper. The chemistry of the porphyrin molecule suggests that this compound should have a greater affinity for copper than for iron. Considerable work is needed to fully assess the relation of copper to porphyrin compounds.

It is apparent that a very close and intimate relationship exists between porphyrins, respiratory enzymes and cerebral function. While the answers are not immediately apparent sufficient evidence exists that hepatic function controls and influences the metabolism of these substances which in turn affect the nervous system.

Lipid Metabolism

More than one half of the aqueous constituents of the brain is lipid composed of cholesterol, cerebrosides, lecithin, cephalin, phospholipids and sphingomyelin. These substances constitute the myelin and are present to some degree in both grey and white matter. The latter is distinguished from the former by the greater concentration of cerebrosides, free cholesterol and sphingomyelin. Johnson, McNabb and Rossiter (408) noted that in infants the lipids were equally distributed in white and grey matter and that they resembled the distribution in the adult cortex. Lipids are also present within neurones and Tyrell and Richter (409) found that the concentration of cerebrosides in the cell nucleus was 100 per cent higher than in the cytoplasm.

It was formerly held that the function of myelin was that of a passive structural one rather than an active metabolic one. However, in recent years through the employment of radioactive tracers of phosphorus and deuterium a cerebral lipid turnover has been demonstrated (401). As a result of this technique the following facts have become known: (1) twenty-four carbon atom fatty acids are characteristic of nerve tissue; (2) the turnover of all cerebral lipids is much greater during the early development of the brain than in the adult in which the lipid turnover is slow and minimal (411); (3) lipids are synthesized within the brain and do not come from other sources. From such facts it would seem that the cerebral lipid metabolism is a relatively independent process. Fisk, Chanutin, and Klingman (412), except for an increase in plasma sphingomyelin, could demonstrate no change in the cerebral lipids in a wide variety of neurological diseases. Crandall and Cherry (413) and Weil and Cleveland (414) noted a lipase in the sera of patients with multiple sclerosis.

Lipid metabolism, to a great extent, is controlled by the liver. This organ regulates the equilibrium between cholesterol and its esters and it is the sole source of body phospholipids which make up part of the myelin, mitochondria and cellular membranes. In hepatic disease the total serum lipids are generally increased (415, 416) but lipid fractions may be decreased. Nova (417) in a study of 21 cases of cirrhosis noted an increase in cerebrosides and a decrease in phospholipids during the advanced stages of the disease. Man, Kartin, Durlacher and Peters (418) found an elevation of the total serum cholesterol and phospholipid in obstructive cirrhosis but in portal cirrhosis and infectious hepatitis, they were reduced.

Pierce and Gofman (419) by means of ultra centrifugation showed greatly elevated blood levels of the Sf 10-20 class lipoproteins suggesting a disturbance of lipoprotein metabolism in acute parenchymal liver disease.

Choline deficient diets are known to cause a disturbance of fat metabolism with an infiltration of fat into the liver. Jervis (420) observed cortical hemorrhages in rats on a choline deficient diet but Foa, Weinstein and Kleppell (421) were unable to demonstrate either cortical hemorrhages or changes in the total lipid, phospholipid or cerebroside content of the brain of animals on this diet.

From such reports it appears that hepatic disease is accompanied by disturbances in fat metabolism but the nature of the impact of this upon cerebral function remains unknown. The importance of phospholipids is emphasized, however, by drawing attention to the fact that the energy required to oxidize glucose within the brain is supplied by phosphate esters particularly adenosine triphosphate and phosphocreatine.

Demyelination is a disturbance of lipid metabolism which occurs in many conditions in addition to hepatic diseases. Many substances are capable of inducing this response in the nervous system and include copper, cyanides, carbon monoxide, nitrous oxide, ether, carbon dioxide, chloroform, arsenic, barbiturates and bile salts, toxins, viruses and antisera, and avitaminosis B (422-

425). Many of these exercise their chief damage on the basal ganglia and according to Hurst (422) the lesion is no different from that produced by the ligation of the large basal brain arteries. Sodium taurocholate and sodium glycocholate, constituents of bile salts, in addition to being hemolysins are also myelinolysins and cause demyelination (426).

Mention has been made of the higher lipid turnover rate of the developing brain compared with that of the adult brain. This process of myelination is intimately related to oxygen consumption since it has been shown by Sperry and Waelsch (427) that the developing brain exhibits a marked increase in oxygen consumption which ceases at the termination of myelination so that the adult rat brain has double the oxygen consumption of the infant one. Myelination is considered to be an oxidative mechanism.

In the adult brain glucose is metabolized to pyruvic and acetic acids the latter burned through the tricarboxylic cycle to carbon dioxide and water with the release of energy (428). In the newborn, oxidation is less and larger amounts of acetic acid are available which are the building stones of fatty acids and cholesterol. A block in this method of lipid synthesis or an increase in lipolytic enzyme is felt to be the cause of demyelination by Sperry and Waelsch (427).

Because of the multiplicity of demyelinating agents it is apparent that all act through a single mechanism which is probably enzymatic in its final analysis. Demyelination is not solely characteristic of hepatic disease but the latter causes changes in chemical and enzymatic equilibria which are capable of causing demyelination.

Bilirubin

The serum bilirubin was elevated in all of the cases presented in Chapter V and all developed hepatic coma. It was mentioned that the serum bilirubin merely reflected the extent of hepatic damage. However, bilirubin may play a much greater role in the production of cerebral symptoms than this. Bilirubin is derived from hemoglobin which is degraded by progressive loss of globin, and ferric chloride so that a cyclic protoporphyrin compound is left. This latter compound when converted to a straight chain is bilirubin, a substance having a molecular weight of 600 and four pyrrol rings (113, 372). It has a great affinity for serum albumin and globulin and is probably conveyed in the blood stream by this means. The chief function of the liver in this regard is the excretion of bilirubin and in the presence of parenchymal failure or duct obstruction, the level of this rises in the blood stream. The effect of bilirubin upon the brain is not known, but it appears in the spinal fluid when the serum bilirubin is elevated over an extended time.

According to Dutlin (429) the infant brain is more permeable and modified bile pigments may be observed in the infant brain or anoxic adult brains. When nuclear masses of the brain are stained with bilirubin the condition is known as kernicterus, not all of which are associated with erythroblastosis foetalis. Hyperbilirubinemia is one prerequisite for kernicterus although the other factors are not clearly understood. The effect of bilirubin on the blood brain barrier has been mentioned.

Hormones

The role of hormones in hepatic dysfunction is not clear but spider naevi, and disturbances in fluid balance are indications of an abnormality of hormone metabolism (323, 329, 325). Mark (329) demonstrated a dissociation between cirrhosis and adrenal cortical function manifest by low urinary excretion of 17 keto-steroids and high cortin excretion. The relation of these factors to the function of the brain has never been studied although this may be advisable in view of the reported effects of cortisone, ACTH and other hormone-like substances on the nervous system and liver. The recent observation of elevated urinary aldosterone in cirrhosis provokes the question as to the role of this substance as a factor in the cerebral symptomatology (430).

Vitamin E

Vitamin E is a substance which exerts a considerable effect on nerve tissue and whose metabolism is altered in hepatic disease.

Gyorgi (431) and others have produced experimental hepatic lesions with tocopherol deficient diets and have likewise demonstrated the beneficial effect of vitamin E in experimental hepatic necrosis. Einarson (432, 433) has studied the effect of a vitamin E deficiency on the central nervous system and described degeneration of the posterior columns, dorsal rootlets with glial proliferation and Alzheimer cells. The physiology of vitamin E is not completely understood but one of its functions is that of a coenzyme for the formation of high energy phosphate bonds such as phosphocreatine and adenosine triphosphate. The Nissl substance of nerve cells is composed of nucleoproteins and ribonucleic acid and are concerned with the formation of adenosine triphosphate which requires vitamin E. In vitamin E deficiencies the adenosine triphosphate and phosphocreatine values are decreased in the grey substance of the brain and Einarson is of the opinion that avitaminosis E causes chronic hypoxia in nerve cells due to defective phosphorylation. Einarson regards vitamin E as a necessary factor in the liberation of adenylic acid which is important in the ultimate production of acetylcholine. This relationship can be expressed in the following equation:

vitamin E + oxygen → adenylic acid + acetyl phosphate → adenosine triphosphate (ATP) → ATP + K (potassium) + acetyl + choline → acetyl choline. The latter substance is well known as a factor in synaptic transmission.

Zinc Metabolism

The role of zinc in cirrhosis has been studied recently by Vallee, Wacker and Bartholomay (434) and Vallee (435), who recorded a decrease in serum zinc levels. Zinc was shown to be present in the enzyme carbonic anhydrase. Glutamic dehydrogenase is a zinc metallo-enzyme which catalyzes the release of ammonia from glutamic acid which is thereby transformed into alpha-keto glutaric acid. Low serum zinc concentration may aid in the accumulation of ammonia whose importance has been discussed. A speculative explanation for the high blood ammonia levels in cirrhosis is offered in light of this information.

Bile salts

Carey (436) has recently made a study of bile salts and noted an increased serum concentration in hepatic disease. In a study of 70 jaundiced patients, 12 of whom had severe liver damage, the ratio between the trihydroxy and dihydroxy bile acids was less than one, due mostly to a five-fold increase in the latter type. Chiefly because of their physical properties the bile salts have been shown to inhibit various enzyme systems. Hockenhull (437) demonstrated a diminished O_2 uptake due to inhibition of succinic dehydrogenase. Ashmore and Nesbett (438) showed that bile acids greatly influence the activity of glucose-6-phosphatase which catalyzes glucose-6-phosphate to glucose. The reaction may be one of inhibition or activation depending upon the substrate and the authors suggest that one substance therefore can regulate the whole enzymatic system. High concentrations of bile acids sufficient to dissolve the cell microsomes will result in loss of enzyme activity. Mann (439) has shown an inhibition of ATPase activity by bile and bile salts. The hydrolysis of glycerol phosphate and hexosphosphate by alkaline phosphatase is inhibited by bile acids according to Takata (440). Evidence also exists for the disturbance of cytochrome oxidase as reported by Eichel, Wainio, and Person (441). The role of bile salts in aiding the penetration of the BBB has been mentioned in an earlier paragraph. The bile salt and acids have previously been dismissed by most investigators as a factor in brain-liver relationships. It would seem that some reconsideration of the role of the bile as a factor in the production of symptoms is necessary.

Vitamin B_{12}

Vitamin B_{12} has been shown by Gyorgy (431), McCormack and Drill (442) to exert a beneficial effect on experimentally produced cirrhosis and it is a lipotropic agent which will defat a fatty liver. Alexander and Backlar (443) have recently related this substance to the genesis of ribonucleoproteins. A thirty-fold increase in vitamin B_{12} serum levels in coma has been demonstrated by Jones and Mills (444). The significance of these facts is not known.

Mechanical Factors

Mechanical factors in hepatic disease may play a role in the production of cerebral changes. Sherlock (445) has demonstrated an increased pressure in the right auricle in cirrhosis which one might expect would compromise the venous return from the cranial cavity and so aid in the development of cerebral edema.

These, then are some of the relationships that exist between the liver and the brain. Many facts are known about hepatic and cerebral functions but the exact sequence of events is not clear. It becomes increasingly apparent that no single factor is the cause of the cerebral change but that multiple metabolic defects may exist together or that one may precede another. In the normal individual nature has created a balanced system with some degree of latitude. The liver is a major organ that is positioned so as to be able to modify, convert or reject any substance absorbed from the gastrointestinal tract. When such an organ with many functions is damaged, not one but several, metabolic cycles are disrupted and the nice balance of nature profoundly disturbed. It is difficult to say which of the many abnormal metabolites conveyed to the nerve tissue in the circulation is the primary or the secondary one. This may be likened to the structure of an atom in which the brain is represented by the nucleus and the body metabolites as electrons in their respective orbits. An abnormality of one value, for example, cytochrome would be represented in this scheme by a change in the orbital relationship of one electron to another which, of course, would disrupt the entire function of the atom.

The brain is bathed in a solution which contains abnormal quantities of bilirubin, bile salts, lipids, iron, copper, globulins, enzymes, cytochromes, phosphorous compounds, albumin, vitamins, prophyrins and perhaps some substances not yet known.

In view of such a number of intricate and intimately related metabolites, it would be foolish to implicate one substance as the cause of the cerebral manifestations of hepatic disease. One can only speculate at this time and the large number of theories advanced so far attests to the large number of possibilities. In the final analysis, one might say with relative impunity that the cell dies because of some interference with its oxygen supply. Innumerable chemical reactions occur between the initial and the terminal stages of oxygen lack. It would seem that enzymatic dysfunction would be most likely the cause of the cerebral change.

SUMMARY AND CONCLUSIONS

A clinical analysis of 42 patients with hepatic disease and coma, of 40 patients with hepatic disease without coma, a clinical classification, and a discussion of some of the relationships that exist between the liver and brain have been presented in this monograph. These studies have indicated that a polybiochemical hepatic disturbance underwrites the polysystemic cerebral involvement in hepatic coma and lesser degrees of brain dysfunction. It would seem, therefore, that no single substance can be incriminated as the cause of the cerebral alterations. This is the chief conclusion to be drawn from this study. We must, therefore, devote our energies to a study of the effects of combinations of abnormalities rather than pursue, hopelessly, one substance. It is to be hoped that this monograph will signal the termination to the era of light microscopy, and clinical correlative studies that have plagued this relationship for decades. The future now demands intensive biochemical study of enzymes, metallo-enzymes, chromogens, bilirubins, cytochromes and metals. Newer liver function studies are needed as well as better tests of brain dysfunction. Further pursuance of correlative studies employing current liver and brain tests, symptoms and signs is futile and let us bury ignominiously the arguments that have existed over the pathological changes observed in the brain for life can scarcely be studied through an appraisal of the dead.

Let us bring into this relationship new ideas, new instruments, new techniques and new measurements so that we may have within the next 10 years the answers, which have eluded us for the past 100 years.

REFERENCES

1. ADAMS, F.: *The Genuine Works of Hippocrates.* New York, Wood, 1886.
2. SINGER, C.: *The Evolution of Anatomy,* Kegan Paul, Trench, Trubner and Company, Ltd., 1925.
3. *Ibid.*
4. GLISSONI, FRANCISI: *Anatomia Hepatis.* Amsterdam, 1659.
5. RUBEOUS, F.: *De Ictero Leth. Noct. Exercit.* 1660, p. 195, after Ozanam.
6. MORGAGNI, G.: *De Sedibus et Causis Morborum.* 1761, translated by Alexander, London.
7. GRIFFIN, W.: On what marked state does the occurrence of coma and sudden death in jaundice depend? *London Med. Gaz., 13:*801, 1834.
8. ALDIS, C. J. B.: Case of jaundice with cerebral affection terminating fatally. *Lond. Med. Gaz., 13:*833, 1834.
9. BRIGHT, R.: Observation on jaundice. *Guy's Hosp. Rep., 1:*604, 1836.
10. BUDD, G.: *Diseases of the Liver.* London, 1845.
11. FRERICHS, F. T.: *A Clinical Treatise on Diseases of the Liver,* Vol. 1. London, New Sydeham Soc., 1860, p. 241.
12. SCHIFF, Prof.: On a new function of the liver. *Med. Times and Gazette,* London, 1877.
13. WESTPHAL, C.: Ueber ime dem Bilde der Cerebrospinalen grauen Degeneration ahnliche Erkranhung des centralen Nervensystems ohne anatomisches Befund nebst imigen Bermerkungen uber paradoxe contraction. *Arch. Psychiat, 14:*87, 1883.
14. LEYDEN, E.: *Beitrage zur Pathologie des Icterus.* Berlin, A. Hirschwald, 1866.
15. GOWERS, W.: *Diseases of the Nervous System,* Vol. 2. London, 1888, p. 656.
16. GOWERS, W.: On tetanoid chorea and its association with cirrhosis of the liver. *Rev. Neurol. and Psychiat., 4:*249, 1906.
17. HOMEN, E. A.: Eine eigenthumliche Familienkrankheit unter der Form liver progressive Dimentia mit besonderen anatomischen Gefund, *Zentralbl. Neurol., 9:*514, 1890.
18. *Ibid.* "Eine eigenthumliche bei drei Geschwistern auftretende typische Krankheit unter der Form einer progressiven Dementia, in Verbindung mit ausgedehunten Gefasserveränderungen (wohl Lues hereditaria tarda)." *Arch. Psychiat., 24:*191, 1892.
19. ORMEROD, J. A.: Cirrhosis of the liver in a boy with obscure and fatal nervous symptoms. *St. Barth. Hosp. Rep., 26:*57, 1890.
20. VON RECKLINGHAUSEN, F.: Uber hemochromatose. *Naturf. n Aerzte, 62:*324, 1889.
21. STRÜMPELL, A.: Ueber die Westphalsche Pseudosklerose und ueber diffuse hirusklerose, inbesondere bei Kindern. *Deutsch. Zentralbl. Nervenh., 12:*115, 1898.
22. FLEISCHER, V.: Die periphere braun-grunlich Hornhauterfarbung als Symptom einer eigenartigen Allgemeinerkrankung. *Munch. med. Wchnschr., 56:*1120, 1909.

23. FLEISCHER, B.: Ueber eine der "Pseudosklerose" nahestehende bisher um-
bekannte Krankheit, gekennzeichnet durch Tremor, psychiche Storung,
braunliche Pigmentierung bestimater Gewebe, insbesondere auch der
Harnhaut peripherie, Lebercirrhose, *Deutsch. Ztschr. Nervenh.*, 64:174,
1912.

24. KAYSER, B.: Ueber einen Fall von angeharner grunlicher Verforbung der
cornea. *Klinische Monatschrift. Augenh.*, 40:22, 1902.

25. ANTON, G.: Dementia chorea-asthenica mit juveniler knotiger Hyperplasia
der Leber. *Munch. med. Wchnscher.*, 46:2369, 1908.

26. WILSON, S. A. K.: Progressive lenticular degeneration: A familial nervous
disease associated with cirrhosis of the liver. *Brain*, 34:295, 1912.

27. WILSON, S. A. K.: *Neurology*, Vol. II. Baltimore, Williams & Wilkins, 1940.

28. POTTS, C. S., and SPILLER, W. G.: Pseudo-Sclerosis (Diffuse Sclerosis),
J.A.M.A., 45: 1455, 1905.

29. GREENFIELD, J. G., POYNTON, F. J., and WALSH, F. M. R.: Progressive
lenticular degeneration. *Quart. J. Med.*, 17:385, 1924.

30. DENNEY-BROWN, D.: *Diseases of the Basal Ganglia and Subthalamic Nuclei*.
Oxford Med. Publications, 1946.

31. HÖSSLIN, C., and ALZHEIMER, A.: Ein Beitrag zur Klinik und pathologischen
Anatomie der Westphal-Strümpell'schen Pseudosklerose. *Ztschr. ges.
Neurol. u. Psychiat.*, 8:183, 1912.

32. LUTHY, F.: Über die hepato-lentikulare Degeneration (Wilson-Westphal-
Strümpell). *Deutsche Ztschr. Nervenh.*, 123:101, 1931.

33. CAMPBELL, C. M., and MORSE, M. E.: A case of Westphal-Strümpell
Pseudosclerosis following erysipelas with a discussion of allied conditions.
J. Neurol. and Psychopath., 5:27, 1924.

34. Hall, H. C.: *La Degenerescence Hepatolenticulaire*. Paris, Masson, 1921.

35. BARNES, S., and HURST, E. W.: Hepatolenticular degeneration, a final note.
Brain, 52:2, 1929.

36. BARNES, S., and HURST, E. W.: Hepatolenticular degeneration. *Brain*,
48:279, 1925.

37. SPIELMEYER, W.: Die histopathologische Zusammengehorigkiet der Wilsonschen Krankheit and der Pseudosklerose. *Ztschr. ges. Neurol. u. Psychiat.*,
57:312, 1920.

38. POLLACK, L. I.: The pathology of the nervous system in a case of progressive lenticular degeneration. *J. Nerv. & Ment. Dis.*, 44:401, 1917.

39. BRAMWELL, B.: Familial cirrhosis of the liver: Four cases of acute fatal
cirrhosis of the liver in the same family, the patients being respectively
nine, ten, fourteen and fourteen years of age: Suggested relationship to
Wilson's progressive degeneration of the lenticular nucleus, *Edinburg
M.J.*, 17:90, 1916.

40. KEHRER, F.: Bemerkungen zu der Arbeit von J. L. Entres: "Genealogische
Studien zur Differential-diagnose zwischen Wilsonscher Krankheit und
Huntingtonscher Chorea." *Ztschr. ges. Neurol. u. Psychiat.*, 100:476, 1926.

41. JENDRALSKI, F.: Der Fleischersche Ring bei Wilsonische Krankheit: Klinischer und anatomischer Beitrog nebst Bermerkungen über den Homo-
siderinring beim Keratokonns. *Klin. Monatsbl. Augenh.*, 68:750, 1922.

42. KRAUPA, E.: Zu Fleischers grunlicher Hornhautverfarbung. *Klin. Monatsbl. Augenh., 69*:526, 1922.

43. HADFIELD, G.: On hepato-lenticular degeneration, with the account of a case and the pathologic findings. *Brain, 46*:11, 1923.

44. BORBERG, N. C.: Ein Fall von Lentikular und Hinterstrangs-degeneration bei adenocarcinom pancreatis mit heparmetastases. *Acta psychiat neurol., 2*:201, 1927.

45. BABONNIEX, L., and WIDIEZ, A.: Choree chronique: Cirrhose avec adenome du foie. *Rev. neurol., 34*:690, 1927.

46. LOWY, J.: Zur Casinstik der Wilson'schen Krankheit. *Deutsches Arch. Klin. Med., 141*: 213, 1922.

47. BROUWER, B.: The spleen, the liver and the brain. *Proc. Roy. Soc. Med., 29*:579, 1936.

48. WAGGONER, R. W., and MALAMUD, N.: Wilson's disease in light of cerebral changes following ordinary acquired liver disorders. *J. Nerv. & Ment. Dis., 96*:410-423, 1942.

49. THADDEA, S., and OETTEL, H. J.: Isolierte Hemochromatose der Haut bei Morbus Wilson. *Ztschr. ges. Neurol. u. Psychiat., 170*:551, 1940.

50. LEWEY, F., and GOVENS, R.: Hemochromatotic pigmentation of the nervous system. *J. Neuropath. & Exper. Neurol., 1*:129, 1942.

51. NEUMAN, M.: Hemochromatosis of the central nervous system. *J. Neuropath. & Exper. Neurol.,* 7:19, 1948.

52. McDOUGAL, D. B., and ADAMS, R. D.: The Neuropathological Changes in hemochromatosis. *J. Neuropath.,* 9:117, 1950.

53. GLAZEBROOK, A. J.: Wilson's disease. *Edinburg M. J., 52*:83, 1945.

54. CUMINGS, J. N.: The copper and iron content of brain and liver in the normal and hepatolenticular degeneration. *Brain, 71*:410-415, 1948.

55. CUMINGS, J. N.: The effects of BAL in hepatolenticular degeneration, *Brain,* 74:10, 1951.

56. SHELDON, J. H.: The iron content of the tissues in hemochromatosis, with special reference to the brain. *Quart. J. Med., 21*:123, 1927-28.

57. ROLLESTON, H.: *Diseases of the Liver, GB and Bile Ducts,* 2nd Ed. Philadelphia, 1912.

58. WILCOX, W. H.: Lettsomian Lectures on Jaundice with Special reference to types occurring during the war. *Tr. M. Soc. London, 42*:147, 1919.

59. ELLIOT, T. R., and WALSHE, F. M. B.: The Babinski or extensor form of plantar response in toxic states. *Lancet, 1*:65, 1925.

60. ADAMS, R. D., and FOLEY, J. M.: Neurologic changes in the more common types of severe liver disease. *Tr. Am. Neurol. A.,* 74:217, 1949.

61. WALSHE, J. M.: Observation on symptoms and pathogenesis of hepatic coma. *Quart. J. Med.,* 20:421, 1951.

62. LUCKE, B.: The pathology of fatal epidemic hepatitis. *Am. J. Path., 20*:471, 1944.

63. STOKES, J. F., OWENS, J. R., and HOHNES, E. G.: Neurological complications of infectious hepatitis. *Brit. M. J.,* 2:642, 1945.

64. GYSIN, W. M., and COOKE, E. T.: Unusual mental symptoms in a case of hepatolenticular degeneration. *Dis. Nerv. System,* 11:305, 1950.

65. LEIBOWITZ, S., and GORMAN, W. F.: Neuropsychiatric complications of viral hepatitis. *New England J. Med., 246*:932, 1952.

66. HARDY, J. L., and FEEMSTER, R. F.: Infectious hepatitis in Massachusetts, with a review of present knowledge of the disease. *New England J. Med.*, 235:147, 1946.
67. BYRNE, E. A. J., and TAYLOR, G. F.: Outbreak of jaundice with signs in nervous system. *Brit. M. J.*, 1:477, 1945.
68. LESCHER, F. G.: Nervous complications of infective hepatitis. *Brit. M. J.*, 1:554-556, 1944.
69. KÜHNE, DR. W.: Beiträge zur Lehre von Icterus: *Virchows Arch.*, (3rd and 4th part) 14:310, 1858.
70. RAPPOPORT, A. M.: Experimental ischaemia of the liver and hepatic coma, coma, liver injury. *Tr. of 10th Conf. Josiah Macy Foundation*, May 21-22, 1951, p. 146.
71. HAHN, M.; MASSEN, O.; NENCKI, M.; and PAWLOW, J.: Die Eckische Fistel Zwischen der Unteren Hohlvene und der Pfartader und Ihre Folgen fur den Organismus. *Arch. exper. Path. u. Pharmakol.*, 32:161, 1893.
72. FUCHS, A.: Experimentelle Enzephalitis. *Wien. med. Wchnschr.*, 71:709, 1921.
73. BALO, J., and KORPASSY, B.: Encephalitis of dogs with Eck fistula fed on meat diets. *Arch. Path.*, 13:80, 1932.
74. BOLLMAN, J. C., and MANN, F. C.: Physiology of impaired liver. *Ergebuis Physiol.*, 38:445, 1936.
75. DEJONG, H. H.: *Experimental Catatonia*, Baltimore, Williams & Wilkins, 1945.
76. MARKOWITZ, J., RAPPOPORT, A. M., and SCOTT, A. C.: The function of the hepatic artery in the dog. *Am. J. Digest. Dis.*, 16:344, 1949.
77. FRASER, D., RAPPOPORT, A. M., VUYLSTEHE, C. A., and COLWELL, A. R., JR.: Effects of ligation of the hepatic artery in dogs. *Surgery*, 30:624, 1951.
78. GRINDLAY, J. H., MANN, F. C., and BOLLMAN, J. L.: Effect of occlusion of the arterial blood supply to the normal liver. *Arch. Surg.*, 62:806, 1951.
79. CRANDALL, L. A., and WEIL, A.: Pathology of central nervous system in diseases of the liver: Experiments with animals and human material. *Arch. Neurol. & Psychiat.*, 29:1066, 1933.
80. EDSALL, D., and DRINKER, C.: The clinical aspects of chronic manganese poisoning. *Contrib. Research*, 1:447, 1919.
81. MELLA, H.: The experimental production of basal ganglion symptomatology in macacus rhesus. *Arch. Neurol. & Psychiat.*, 11:405, 1924.
82. WILLIAMSON, C. S., and MANN, F. C.: Studies on the physiology of the liver. The hepatic factor in chloroform and phosphorous poisoning. *Am. J. Physiol.*, 65:267, 1923.
83. MALLORY, F. B.: The relation of chronic poisoning with copper to hemochromatosis. *Am. J. Path.*, 1:117, 1925.
84. HURST, E. W., and HURST, P. E.: The aetiology of hepato-lenticular degeneration. Experimental liver cirrhosis. Poisoning with manganese chloroform, phenylhydrozine, bile and guanidin. *J. Path. and Bact.*, 31:303, 1928.
85. HOFFBAUER, F. W.: Personal communication.
86. GYORGY, P.: Experimental hepatic injury. *Am. J. Clin. Path.*, 14:67, 1944.

87. HIMSWORTH, H. P., and GLYNN, L. E.: Massive hepatic necrosis and diffuse hepatic fibrosis (acute yellow atrophy and portal cirrhosis): Their production by means of diet. *Clin. Sc.,* 5:93, 1944.

88. HARTROFT, W. S.: Histologic studies on fatty infiltration of the liver in choline-deficient rats, in Ciba Foundation Symposium, *Liver Disease,* Philadelphia, Blakiston, 1951, p. 90.

89. CHESNEY, A. M., MARSHALL, E. K., and ROWNTREE, L. G.: Studies in liver function. *J.A.M.A.,* 63:1533, 1914.

90. STADIE, W. C., and VAN SLYKE, D. D.: The effect of acute yellow atrophy on metabolism and on the composition of the liver. *Arch. Int. Med.,* 25:693, 1920.

91. UZMAN, L., and BROWN, D. DENNY: Aminoaciduria in hepato-lenticular degeneration (Wilson's disease). *Am. J. M. Sc.,* 215:599, 1948.

92. DENT, C. E., and WALSHE, J. M.: Amino acid metabolism in liver disease, in *Liver Disease,* Ciba, Symposium. Philadelphia, Blakiston, 1951, p. 22.

93. DEVERDIER, C.: Paper chromatographic analysis of amino acid excretion in Wilson's disease. *Acta. med. scandinav.,* 138:344, 1950.

94. COOPER, A. M., ECKHARDT, R. O., FALOON, W. W., and DAVIDSON, C. S.: Investigation of aminoaciduria in Wilson's disease: Demonstration of defect in renal function. *J. Clin. Investigation,* 29:265, 1950.

95. ROMAN, B.: Acute yellow atrophy of the liver. *Arch. Path.,* 4:399, 1927.

96. QUASTEL, J. H.: Enzymic activity of the brain. *Proc. Roy. Soc. Med.,* (Part 1) 29:200, 1935.

97. WEIL, A., and MALHERBE, H.: XCV. Studies on brain metabolism, 1. The metabolism of glutamic acid in brain. *Biochem. J.,* 30:665, 1936.

98. AMATUZIO, D. S., and NESBITT, S.: A study of pyruvic acid in the blood spinal fluid and urine of patients with liver disease with and without hepatic coma. *J. Clin. Investigation,* 29:796, 1950.

99. SNELL, A. M., and BUTT, H. R.: Hepatic coma; observations bearing on its nature and treatment, *Tr. Am. Physicians,* 56:321, 1941.

100. PLANER, J.: Ueber das Varkommen von Pigment im Blute. *Stschr. Gesellschaft Aerzte Wien,* 10:127, 280, 1854.

101. BOENHEIM, F.: Beitrog zur Kenntnis der Pseudosklerose und Verwandter Krankheiten unter Besonderer Berucksichtigung der Beziehung Zwischen den Erkrankungen des Gehirns und der Leber. *Ztschr. ges Neurol. u. Psychiat.,* 60:10, 1920.

102. NAYRAC, P.: Considerations nosologiques et pathogeniques sur la degenerescence hepato-lenticulaire. *Rev. neurol.,* 2:151, 1924.

103. OBERLING, C., and KALBO, A.: Troubles circulatoires au foie consecutifs a des lesions experimentales des noyaux, gris centraux. *Compt. rend. Soc. biol.,* 102:916, 1929.

104. CROFTAN, A. C.: Hepatic insufficiency: Its causes, recognition, significance and treatment. *M. Rec.,* 69:653-656, 1906.

105. BAKER, A. B.: The central nervous system in hepatic disease. *J. Neuropath. & Exper. Neurol.,* 8:283, 1949.

196. LEIGH, A. D., & CARD, W. I.: Hepato-lenticular degeneration. A case associated with posterolateral column degeneration. *J. Neuropath. & Exper. Neurol.,* 8:338, 1949.

107. MASON, E. C., and DAVIDSON, E. C.: A study of tissue autolysis in vivo. II: A pharmacological study of the toxic material. *J. Lab. & Clin. Med.,* 10:906-913, 1925.

108. HEYD, C. G.: The concept of liver deaths. *J.A.M.A., 121*:736, 1943.

109. SCHILLER, O.: Disturbance of Liver Function Causing Cerebral Changes, *Wien. klin. Wchnschr., 61*:751, 1949.

110. BIELSCHOWSKY, M., and HALLERVORDEN, J.: Symmetrische Einschmelzungsherde im Stirnhirn beim Wilson-Pseudosklerose Komplex. *J. Psychol. u. Neurol., 42*:177, 1931.

111. ROSSLE, R.: Entzundungen der Leber. *Hand. Spez. path. Anat. u. Histol.,* 5:462, 1930.

112. SCHIFF, L.: *Diseases of the Liver.* Philadelphia, Lippincott, 1956.

113. LICHTMAN, S. S.: *Diseases of the Liver, Gallbladder and Bile Duets.* Philadelphia, Lea, 1953.

114. SHERLOCK, S.: *Diseases of the Liver and Biliary System,* Oxford, Blackwell; Springfield, Thomas, 1955.

115. KNISELY, M. H.: *Tr. Tenth Conf. Liver Injury.* Jos. Macy Jr. Foundation, 1951, p. 48.

116. LESCHKE, E.: Ueber die Gelbfährung (Xanthochromic) der Zerebrospinalflussigkeit. *Leutsche med. Wchnschr., 47*:376, 1921.

117. HIMSWORTH, H. P.: *Lectures on the Liver and Its Disease.* Cambridge, Harvard, 1947.

118. WATSON, C. J., and HOFFBAUER, F. W.: Liver function in hepatitis. *Ann. Int. Med., 26*:813, 1947.

119. POPPER, H., STEIGMAN, F., MEYER, K. A., KOZOLL, D. D., and FRANKLIN, M.: Correlation of liver function and liver structure; clinical applications. *Am. J. Med., 6*:278, 1949.

120. HOFFBAUER, F. W.: Coproporphyrin excretion in experimental liver injury. *J. Clin. Investigation, 29*:822, 1950.

121. WATSON, C. J., SUTHERLAND, D., and HAWKINSON, V.: Studies of coproporphyrin. V. The isomer distribution and per diem excretion of the urinary coproporphyrin in cases of cirrhosis of the liver. *J. Lab. & Clin. Med., 37*:1, 1951.

122. WATSON, C. J., HAWKINSON, V., CAPPS, R. B., and RAPPOPORT, E. M.: Studies of coproporphyrin IV. The perdiem excretion and isomer distribution in the urine in infectious hepatitis, infectious mononucleosis and mechanical jaundice. *J. Clin. Investigation, 28*:621, 1949.

123. POPPER, H., de la Duerga, J., Steigmann, F., and Sladki, M.: Turbidimetric gamma globulin determinations in hepatobiliary diseases, *J. Lab. & Clin. Med., 35*:391, 1950.

124. SPELLBERG, M. A., COHN, C., WOLFSON, W. Q., and SHORE, C.: Serum globulin fractions as an index of hepatic dysfunction. *Gastroenterology,* 14:11, 1950.

125. MARRACK, J. R., and HOCH, H.: Serum proteins: A review, *J. Clin. Path.,* 2:161, 1949.

126. MACLAGEN, N. F.: Thymol turbidity test, an indication of liver dysfunction. *Brit. J. Exper. Path., 25*:234, 1944.

127. COHEN, P. P., and THOMPSEN, F. L.: Mechanisms of the thymol turbidity test, *J. Lab. Clin. & Med., 32*:475, 1947.

128. Hanger, F. M.: Serological differentiation of obstructive from hepatogenous jaundice by flocculation of cephalin cholesterol emulsions. *J. Clin. Investigation, 18*:261, 1939.

129. Watson, C. J., and Rappoport, E. M.: A comparison of the results obtained with the hanger cephalin cholesterol flocculation test and the MacLagen thymol turbidity test in patients with liver disease. *J. Lab. & Clin. Med., 30*:983, 1945.

130. Frerichs, F. T.: *Über den Diabetes,* Berlin, 1884.

131. Zamcheck, N., and Sidman, R. L.: Needle biopsy of the liver: I. Its use in clinical and investigative medicine. *New England J. Med., 249*:1020, 1953.

132. McCartney, J. S.: *In Textbook of Pathology,* E. T. Bell, ed. Philadelphia, Lea, 1947, p. 573.

133. Josselin De Jong, R.: Lebercirrhose. *Compt. rend. Conf. Internat. Path. Geogr.,* p. 38, 1931.

134. Kretz, R.: Cirrhosis of the liver. *Internat. Clin., 15*:289, 1905.

135. Mann, F. C., and Magath, T. B.: The production of chronic liver insufficiency, *Am. J. Physiol., 59*:485, 1922.

136. Fishback, F. C.: Morphologic study of regeneration of liver after partial removal. *Arch. Path., 7*:955, 1929.

137. Higgins, G. M., and Anderson, R. M.: Experimental pathology of the liver I. Restoration of the liver of the white rat following partial surgical removal, *Arch. Path., 12*:180, 1931.

138. Brues, A. M., Drury, D. R., and Brues, M. C.: A quantitative study of cell growth in regenerating liver. *Arch. Path. 22*:658, 1936.

139. Kelty, R. H., Baggenstoss, A. H., and Butt, H. R.: Relation of regenerated liver nodule to vascular bed in cirrhosis. *Gastroenterology, 15*:285, 1950.

140. McIndoe, A. H.: Vascular lesions of portal cirrhosis. *Arch. Path. and Lab. Med., 5*:23, 1928.

141. MacCallum, W. G.: Regenerative changes in cirrhosis of the liver. *J.A.M.A., 43*:649, 1904.

142. Beaver, D. C., and Robertson, H. E.: The specific character of toxic cirrhosis as observed in cincophen poisoning. *Am. J. Path., 7*:237, 1931.

143. Moon, V. H.: Experimental cirrhosis in relation to human cirrhosis, coma; clinical and laboratory observations on 40 patients, *New England J. Med., 239*:605, 1948.

144. Murphy, T. L., Chalmers, T. C., Eckhardt, R. O., and Davidson, C. S.: Hepatic coma; clinical and laboratory observations on 40 patients. *New England J. Med., 239*:605, 1948.

145. Gibson, W. R., and Robertson, H. E.: Obstructive biliary cirrhosis. *Arch. Path., 78*:37, 1939.

146. Hartroft, W. S., and Ridout, J. H.: Pathogenesis of the cirrhosis produced by choline deficiency: Escape of lipid from fatty hepatic cysts into the biliary and vascular systems. *Am. J. Path., 27*:951, Nov.-Dec. 1951.

147. Rich, A. R., and Hamilton, J. D.: The experimental production of cirrhosis of the liver by means of a deficient diet. *Bull. Johns Hopkins Hosp., 66*:185, 1940.

148. Chaikoff, I. L., Conner, C. L., and Biskind, G. R.: Fatty infiltration and

cirrhosis of the liver in depancreatized dogs maintained with insulin. *Am. J. Path.,* 14:101, 1938.

149. CHAIKOFF, I. L., EICHORN, K. B., CONNER, C. L. and ENTENMAN, C.: The production of cirrhosis in the liver of the normal dog by prolonged feeding of a high fat diet. *Am. J. Path.,* 19:9, 1943.

150. BJORNEBOE, M.: Etiology of hepatic cirrhosis. Ciba Symposium, *Liver Disease,* 1952, p. 109.

151. RUNYAN, J., WRIGHT, A. W., and BEEBE, R. T.: Homologous serum jaundice: Report of 8 fatal cases. *J.A.M.A.,* 144:1065, 1950.

152. WATSON, C. J.: Discussion on Experimental ischaemia of the liver and hepatic coma, by Rappoport, A. M. *Liver Injury.* Tr. 10th Conference, Josiah Macy Foundation, 1951, p. 165.

153. PALMER, E. D., and BRICK, I. B.: Esophageal varices in non-cirrhotic patients. *Am. J. Med.,* 17:641, 1954.

154. FAGIN, I. D., and THOMPSON, F. M.: Cirrhosis of the liver: Analysis of 71 cases. *Ann. Int. Med.,* 21:285, 1944.

155. LOGAN, A. H.: Chronic ulcerative colitis. A review of 117 cases. *Northwest. Med.,* 18:1, 1919.

156. COMFORT, M. W., BARGEN, J. A., and MORLOCK, C. G.: The association of chronic ulcerative colitis with hepatic insufficiency: Report of 4 cases. *M. Clin. North America,* 22:1089, 1938.

157. CAIN, A., and CATTAN, R.: Le role de l'hepatite degenerative graisseuse dans l'evolution et le prognostic des rectocolites suppurees. *Soc. med. hôp Paris,* 17:673, 1937.

158. JONES, W. G., BAGGENSTOSS, A. H., and BORGEN, J. A.: Hepatic lesions and dysfunction associated with chronic ulcerative colitis. *Am. J. M. Sc.,* 221:279, 1951.

159. POPPER, H., and SCHAFFNER, F.: Laboratory diagnosis of liver disease, coordinated use of histological and biochemical observations. *J.A.M.A., 150*: 1367, 1952.

160. POPPER, H., WALDSTEIN, S. S., and SZANTO, P. B.: Correlation of clinical features of cirrhosis of the liver with findings on biopsy. *Am. J. Clin. Path.,* 20:724, 1950.

161. SHERLOCK, S. P. V.: Biochemical investigation in liver disease, some correlations with hepatic histology. *J. Path. & Bact.,* 58:523, 1946.

162. POPPER, H., STEIGMANN, F., and SZANTO, P. B.: Quantitative correlation of morphologic liver changes and clinical tests. *Am. J. Clin. Path.,* 19:710, 1949.

163. HOFFBAUER, F. W., EVANS, G. T., and WATSON, C. J.: Cirrhosis of the liver with particular reference to correlation of composite liver function studies with liver biopsy. *M. Clin. North America,* p. 363, 1945.

164. KINSELL, L. W., WEISS, H. A., MICHAELS, G. D., SHAVER, J. C., and BARTON, H. C.: The correlation of hepatic structure and function. *Am. J. Med.,* 6:292, 1949.

165. BEAN, W. B.: Note on the development of cutaneous arterial spiders and palmar erythema in persons with liver disease and their development following administration of estrogens. *Am. J. M. Sc.,* 204:251, 1942.

166. SHERLOCK, S., SUMMERSKILL, W. H. J., WHITE, L. P., and PHEAR, E. A.;

Portal-systemic encephalopathy. Neurological complications of liver disease. *Lancet,* 267:453, 1954.

167. SHERLOCK, S.: Portal-systemic encephalopathy in liver disease. *Proc. Roy. Soc. Med.,* 48:479, 1955.

168. KLINKOVA-DEUTSCHOVA, E. Z.: Neurologicke komplikace hepatitis epidemica. *Z. Neurol. Klin. Praha,* 56:25, 1954.

169. SHERLOCK, S., CULVER, P. J., CASTLEMAN, B., ADAMS, R. D., McDERMOTT, W. V., and AUSTEN, F. K.: Hepatic coma and ammonia metabolism, medical grand rounds, Massachusetts General Hosp. *Am. Pract.,* 7:801, 1956.

170. CAMERON, J. D. S.: Infective hepatitis. *Quart. J. Med.,* 36:139, 1943.

171. SPENCE, J. C., and OGILVIE, A. G.: Cholemia, clinical study of nervous symptom in liver atrophy. *Arch. Dis. Childhood,* 2:41, 1927.

172. DOZARETS, Y. L., and BELOUSOVA, V.: Neurological and psychiatric lesions in acute hepatitis. *Klin. med.,* 10:56, 1950.

173. HOURAL, V.: Neurological complications in epidemic hepatitis. *Cas. Lek ces,* 89:1402, 1950.

174. ZIMMERMAN, H. J., and LOWRY, C. F.: Encephalomyeloradiculitis (Guillain-Barre syndrome) as complication of infectious hepatitis. *Ann. Int. Med.,* 26:934, 1947.

175. SEPULVEDA, B., and PENICHE, J. H.: Acute myelitis probably secondary to viral hepatitis; case report. *Riv. Invest. Clinica Neurio.,* 1:375, 1949.

176. REHM, C. C., and BROCK, W. M.: Acute infectious hepatitis; case associated with Guillain-Barre syndrome. *Northwest. Med.,* 45:343, 1946.

177. WEINSTEIN, L., and DAVISON, W. T.: Neurologic manifestations in infectious hepatitis. *Am. Pract.,* 1:191, 1946.

178. COOPER, G. R.: Paper electrophoretic studies of serum proteins in viral hepatitis. *Am. J. Med.,* 19:646, 1955.

179. SCHAFFNER, F., SCHERBEL, A. L., and LYTLE, R. I.: Serum glycoproteins in viral hepatitis. *Am. J. Med.,* 19:646, 1955.

180. MARTIN, N. H., and DAVIES, H.: Hyperglobulinemia in hepatitis. *Lancet,* 269: 1011, 1955.

181. BERMAN, L. B., LAPHAM, L. W., and PASTORE, E.: Jaundice and xanthochromia in the spinal fluid. *J. Lab. & Clin. Med.,* 44:273, 1954.

182. CARDON, L., and ATLAS, D. H.: Incidence and causes of hyperproteinemia, A study of 4390 cases. *Arch Int. Med.,* 71:377, 1943.

183. BING, J., and NEEL, A. V.: Two cases of hyperglobulinemia with affection of the central nervous system on a toxi-infectious basis. *Acta med. scandinav.,* 88:492, 1936.

184. BING, J., and NEEL, A. V.: Report of a third case of hyperglobulinemia with affection of the central nervous system on a toci-infectious basis. *Acta med. scandinav.,* 91:409, 1937.

185. GUSTAD, V.: Transient hepatargy. *Acta med. scandinav.,* 135:354, 1949.

186. McDERMOTT, W., and ADAMS, R. D.: Eck-fistula—A cause of episodic stupor in humans. *J. Clin. Investigation,* 32:587, 1953.

187. NESBITT, S.: Excretion of coproporphyrin in hepatic disease. III. Urinary excretion of coproporphyrin in hepatic insufficiency during episodes characterized by neurological manifestations. *Arch. Int. Med.,* 71:62, 1943.

188. McDermott, W. V., Wareham, J., and Riddell, A. G.: Treatment of "Hepatic coma" with 1-glutamic acid. *New England J. Med., 253*:1093, 1955.

189. Skinner, H. A.: *The Origin of Medical Terms.* Baltimore Williams & Wilkins, 1949.

190. Adams, R. D., and Foley, J. M.: The neurological disorder associated with liver disease in metabolic and toxic diseases of the nervous system. *A. Res. Nerv. & Ment. Dis., Proc. 32*:1953.

191. LePage, G. A.: Effects of hemorrhage on tissue metabolites. *Am. J. Physiol., 147*:446, 1946.

192. Foley, J. M., Watson, C. W., and Adams, R. D.: Significance of the electroencephalographic changes in hepatic coma. *Tr. Am. Neurol. A.*, p. 161. 1950.

193. Bickford, R. G., and Butt, H. R.: E.E.G. findings in hepatic coma. *Electroencephalog. & Clin. Neurophysiol., 5*:480, 1953.

194. McDermott, W. V., Jr., and Adams, R. D.: Episodic stupor associated with an Eck-fistula in the human with particular reference to the metabolism of ammonia. *J. Clin. Investigation, 33*:1, 1954.

195. Riddell, A. G., and McDermott, W. V.: Hepatic coma. *Lancet, 266*:1263, 1954.

196. Whitfield, A. G. W., and Arnott, W. M.: Transient disturbance of consciousness in hepatic cirrhosis. *Brit. M. J., 2*:1054, 1951.

197. Walshe, J. M.: The effect of glutamic acid on the coma of hepatic failure. *Lancet, 1*:1075, 1953.

198. Ducci, H., and Katz, R.: Cortisone, ACTH and antibiotics in fulminant hepatitis. *Gastroenterology, 21*:357, 1952.

199. Goldbloom, R. S., and Steigmann, F.: Aureomycin therapy in hepatic insufficiency. *Gastroenterology, 18*:93, 1951.

200. Latner, A. L.: Treatment of acute liver disease. *Brit. M. J., 2*:44, 1952.

201. Latner, A. L.: Regime for treatment of severe and acute liver disease, *Brit. M. J., 2*:748, 1950.

202. Kitamura, R.: Experimental studies on the influence of vitamin B complex and of methionine upon liver function. *Jap. Arch. Int. Med., 2*:595, 1955.

203. *Ibid.*: Part II: Effect of vitamin B_6 and of nicotinamide in special reference to comparison with riboflavin. *Jap. Arch. Int. Med., 2*:599, 1955.

204. *Ibid.*: Part III: Effect of Vitamin B_{12} and of Folic Acid. *Jap. Arch. Int. Med., 2*:603, 1955.

205. Najarian, J. S., and Harper, H. A.: A clinical study of the effect of arginine on blood ammonia. *Am. J. Med., 21*:832, 1956.

206. Najarian, J. S., and Harper, H. A.: Comparative effect of arginine and monosodium glutamate on blood ammonia. *Proc. Soc. Exper. Biol. & Med., 92*:560, 1956.

207. Eck, N. V.: On the question of ligature of the portal vein. *Voyenno M.J.* (St. Petersburg) p. 130, 1877.

208. Van Coulaert, C., and Deviller, C.: Ammonieme experimentelle apries ingestion de chlorure d'ammonium chez l'homme a l'état normal et pathologigne. *Compt. rend. Soc. Biol., 111*:50, 1932.

209. Mongiuo, J., and Krause, F.: Über die Bedeutung des NH_3-Gehaltes des

Blutes für die Beurteilung der Leberfunktion: Studien am Normalen Lebergeschadigten und Eckschen Fistethund. *Klin. Wchnschr., 13*:1142, 1934.

210. KIRK, E.: Amino acid and ammonia metabolism in liver disease. *Acta med. scandinav.*, Suppl. 77, 1936.

211. WHITE, L. P., PHEAR, E. A., SUMMERSKILL, W. H. J., SHERLOCK, S., and COLE, M.: Ammonium tolerance in liver disease; observations based on catheterization of the hepatic vein. *J. Clin. Investigation, 34*:158, 1955.

212. BESSMAN, S. P., and BESSMAN, A. N.: The cerebral and peripheral uptake of ammonia in liver disease with an hypothesis for the mechanism of hepatic coma. *J. Clin. Investigation, 34*:622, 1955.

213. SEEGMILLER, J. E., SCHWARTZ, R., and DAVIDSON, C. S.: The plasma "ammonia" and glutamine content in patients with hepatic coma. *J. Clin. Investigation, 33*:984, 1954.

214. TRAEGAR, H. S., GABUZDA, G. J., BALLOU, A. N., and DAVIDSON, C. S.: Blood "ammonia" concentration in liver disease and in liver coma. *Metabolism, 3*:99, 1954.

215. CONWAY, E. J.: *Microdiffusion Analysis and Volumetric Error.* London, Crosby, Lockwood and Son Ltd., 1939.

216. CONWAY, E. J.: Apparatus for the micro-determination of certain volatile substances, IV. The blood ammonia, with observations on normal human blood. *Biochem. J., 29*:2755, 1935.

217. CONWAY, E. J.: *Micro-diffusion Analysis and Volumetric Error,* 3rd Ed. New York, Van Nostrand, 1950.

218. DE GROTTE, J., DESCHEPPER, P., and VANDERBROUCKE, J.: Glutamic acid in hepatic coma. *Lancet, 269*:722, 1955.

219. CHAIKIN, N. W., KONIGSBERG, M. S., and SCHWINIMER, M.: Glutamic acid in hepatic coma. *Am. J. Gastroenterol., 26*:258, 1956.

220. MANN, J. D., BOLLMAN, J. L., HINZENGA, K. A., FARRAR, T., and GRINDLAY, J. H.: Blood ammonia, experimental and clinical study in abnormalities of the liver in portal circulation. *Gastroenterology, 27*:399, 1954.

221. WEBSTER, L. T., and DAVIDSON, C. S.: The effect of sodium glutamate on hepatic coma. *J. Clin. Investigation, 35*:191, 1956.

222. McDERMOTT, W. V., ADAMS, R. D., and RIDDELL, A. G.: Changes in man and animals with portocaval anastomosis. *Proc. Roy. Soc. Med., 48*:481, 1955.

223. GABUZDA, G. J., JR., PHILLIPS, G. B., and DAVIDSON, C. S.: Reversible toxic manifestations in patients with cirrhosis of the liver given cation exchange resins. *N. England J. Med., 246*:124, Jan. 1952.

224. PHILLIPS, G. B., SCHWARTZ, R., GABUZDA, G. J. JR., and DAVIDSON, C. S.: The syndrome of impending hepatic coma in patients with cirrhosis of the liver given certain nitrogenous substances. *New England J. Med., 247*:239, 1952.

225. WEBSTER, L. T., JR., and DAVIDSON, C. S.: Sources of blood ammonium after feeding protein to patients with hepatic cirrhosis. *J. Clin. Investigation. 35*:742, 1956.

226. SUMMERSKILL, W. H., WOLFE, S. J., and DAVIDSON, C. S.: Ammonia intoxication and hepatic coma. *Arch. Int. Med., 97*:661, 1956.

227. FALOON, W. W., AUCHINCLOSS, J., EICH, R., and GILBERT, R.: Ammonia metabolism in cirrhotic patients with portocaval shunts. *J. Clin. Investigation*, 35:701, 1956.

228. WEBSTER, L. T.: Ammonia and coma; American Association Liver Dis. *Lancet*, 269:1322, 1955.

229. BESSMAN, S. P., and BRADLEY, J. E.: Uptake of ammonia by muscle. Its implications in ammoniagenic coma. *New England J. Med.*, 253:1143, 1955.

230. NELSON, R. M., and SELIGSON, D.: Studies on blood ammonia in normal and shock states. *Surgery*, 34:1, 1953.

231. BEATON, J. R., McGANITY, W. J., and McHENRY, E. W.: Plasma glutamic acid levels in malignancy. *Canad. M. A. J.*, 65:219, 1951.

232. WECHSLER, R. L., CRUM, W., and ROTH, J. L. A.: The blood flow and oxygen consumption of the human brain in hepatic coma. *Clin. Research Proc.*, 2:74, 1954.

233. FAZEKAS, J. F., and BESSMAN, A. N.: Quoted by Bessman and Bessman (212).

234. BESSMAN, S. P., and BESSMAN, A. N.: Ammonia poisoning of hepatic coma; Cerebral arteriovenous amino-acid levels. *Federation Proc.*, 13:336, 1954.

235. POTTER, V. R., and RECKNAGEL, R. O.: Alternative metabolic pathways in rat liver homogenates. *Federation Proc.*, 9:215, 1950.

236. SHERLOCK, S., PHEAR, E. A., RUEBNER, B., and SUMMERSKILL, W. H.: Ammonia and coma, American Assoc. Liver Diseases. *Lancet*, 269:1322, 1955.

237. SUMMERSKILL, W. H., SHERLOCK, S., and DAVIDSON, C. S.: Ammonia and coma, American Assoc. Liver Diseases. *Lancet*, 269:1322, 1955.

238. SUMMERSKILL, W. H., DAVIDSON, E. A., SHERLOCK, S., and STEINER, R. E.: The neuropsychiatric syndrome associated with hepatic cirrhosis and intensive portal collateral circulation. *Quart. J. Med.*, 25:245, 1956.

239. HUNT, A. H., and WHITTARD, B. R.: Thrombosis of the portal vein in cirrhosis of the liver. *Lancet*, 266:281, 1954.

240. RUMPEL, A.: Über das Wesen und die Bedeutung der Leber Veranderungen und der Pigmentierungen bei den Damit Verbunden Fallen von Pseudo-sklerose, zugleich ein Beitrag zur Lehre von Pseudosklerose. *Deutsche Ztschr. Nervenh.*, 49:54, 1913.

241. GORDON, A. H., and RABINOWITCH, I. M.: Yellow atrophy of the liver, report of a case with particular reference to the metabolism of copper. *Arch. Int. Med.*, 51:143, 1933.

242. CHERBULIEZ, E., and AUSBACHER, S.: Beitrag zur Bestimmung von Kufer in Organen. *Virchows Arch.*, 278:365, 1930.

243. HERKEL, W.: Über die Bedeutung des Kupfers in der Biologie und Pathologie. *Beitr. path. Anat. u. allg. Path.*, 85:513, 1930.

244. OSHIMA, F., and SCHONHEIMER, R.: Über den Kupfergehalt der normalen Leber und der Leber bei Hamochromatose sowie, von Gallensteinen und Gesamtblut. *Ztschr. physiol. Chem.*, 180:252, 1929.

245. DRY, T. J., Hemochromatosis: Its relation to the metabolism of iron and copper. *Minnesota Med.*, 17:301, 1934.

246. WADDEL, J., STEENBOCK, H., ELVEHJEM, C. A., and HART, E. B.: Iron in nutrition. *J. Biol. Chem.*, 77:769, 1928.

247. HAUROWITZ, F.: Über eine Anomalie des Kupferstoffwechsels. *Ztschr. Physiol. Chem., 190:*72, 1930.

248. PORTER, H.: Copper excretion in urine of normal individuals and of patients with hepatolenticular degeneration (Wilson's disease). *Arch. Biochem, 31:*262, April 1951.

249. BRINTON, O.: Wilson's disease. *Proc. Roy. Soc. Med., 40:*556, Aug. 1947.

250. WARNOCK, C. G.: Hepatolenticular degeneration (Wilson's disease). *Ulster M. J., 21:*155, 1952.

251. ANDRE, M. J.: Des signes biologiques et des caracteres cliniques de la cirrhose Wilsonienne. Leur signification au point de vue de la physiopathologie de la degenerescence lenticulaire. *Rev. belge sc. méd.,* Louvain, *17:*185, 1946.

252. HERZ, E., and DREW, A. L.: Hepatolenticular degeneration. *Arch. Neurol. & Psychiat., 63:*843, 1950.

253. HOMBURGER, F., and KOZOL, H. L.: Hepatolenticular degeneration. *J.A.M.A., 130:*6, 1946.

254. HORNBOSTEL, H.: More recent knowledge concerning hepatolenticular syndrome. *Schweiz. med. Wchnschr., 84:*7, 1954.

255. FRANKLIN, E. C., and BAUMAN, A.: Liver dysfunction in hepatolenticular degeneration, review of 11 cases. *Am. J. Med., 15:*450, 1953.

256. STEPHENS, J. W.: The E.E.G. in hepatolenticular degeneration. *Electroencephalog. & Clin. Neurophysiol., 4:*110, 1952.

257. RAVIN, H. A.: Rapid test for hepatolenticular degeneration. *Lancet, 270:*726, 1956.

258. GUILLAIN, G., BERTRAND, I., and MME. GODET-GUILLAIN: Etude anatomique d'un cas de "syndrome hepato-lenticulaire." Attiente tres accentrice des regions corticale de l'encephale. *Rev. neurol., 90:*169, 1954.

259. MANDELBROTE, B. M., STANIER, M. W., THOMPSON, R. H. S., and THURSTON, M. N.: Studies on copper metabolism in demyelinating diseases of the central nervous system. *Brain, 71:*212, 1948.

260. OKINAKA, S., YOSHIKAWA, M., TOYODA, M., MOZAI, T., TOYOKURA, Y., and KAMEYAMA, M.: Pathogenesis of hepatocerebral disease. *Arch. Neurol. & Psychiat., 72:*573, 1954.

261. CARTWRIGHT, G. E., HODGES, R. E., GUBLER, C. J., MAHONEY, J. P., DAUM, K., WINTROBE, M. M., and BEAN, W. B.: Studies on copper metabolism XIII. Hepatolenticular degeneration. *J. Clin. Investigation, 33:*1487, 1954.

262. MARKOWITZ, H., GUBLER, C. J., MAHONEY, J. P., CARTWRIGHT, G. E., and WINTROBE, M. M.: Studies on copper metabolism XIV: Copper, ceruloplasmin and oxidase activity in sera of normal human subjects, pregnant women, and patients with infection, hepatolenticular degeneration and the nephrotic syndrome. *J. Clin. Investigation, 34:*1498, 1955.

263. MATHEWS, W. B.: The absorption and excretion of radiocopper in hepatolenticular degeneration (Wilson's disease). *J. Neurol., Psychiat. & Neurosurg., 17:*242, 1954.

264. SCHEINBERG, I. H., and GITLIN, D.: Deficiency of ceruloplasmin in patients with hepatolenticular degeneration (Wilson's disease). *Science, 116:*484, 1952.

265. KOREY, F. R., and NURENBERGER, J. I.: *Neurochemistry.* New York, Hoeber-Harper, 1956.

266. SCHEINBERG, I. H., COOK, C. D., and MURPHY, J. A.: The concentration of copper and ceruloplasmin in maternal and infant plasma and delivery. *J. Clin. Investigation, 33*:963, 1954.

267. HAGBERG, B., AXTRUPS, S., and BERFENSTAM, R.: Heavy metals (iron, copper, zinc) in the blood of the foetus and of the infant. *Etudes neo-natales, 2*:81, 1953.

268. LAHEY, M. E., GUBLER, C. J., CARTWRIGHT, G. E., and WINTROBE, M. M.: Studies on copper metabolism. VII. Blood copper in pregnancy and in various pathologic states. *J. Clin. Investigation, 32*:329, 1953.

269. MATHEWS, W. B., MILNE, M. D., and BELL, M.: The metabolic disorder in hepatolenticular degeneration. *Quart. J. Med., 21*:425, 1952.

270. BUSH, J. A., MAHONEY, J. P., MARKOWITZ, H., GUBLER, C. J., CARTWRIGHT, G. E., and WINTROBE, M. M.: Studies on copper metabolism: XVI. Radioactive copper. Studies in normal subjects and in patients with hepatolenticular degeneration. *J. Clin. Investigation, 34*:1766, 1955.

271. DENNY-BROWN, D., and PORTER, H.: The effect of B.A.L. (2, 3-dimercoptopropanol) on hepatolenticular degeneration (Wilson's disease). *New England J. Med., 245*:917, 1951.

272. UZMAN, L. L., and HOOD, B.: The familial nature of the amino-aciduria of Wilson's disease (hepatolenticular degeneration). *Am. J. M. Sci., 223*: 392, 1952.

273. UZMAN, L. L.: On the relationship of urinary copper excretion to the aminoaciduria in Wilson's disease (hepatolenticular degeneration). *Am. J. M. Sc. 226*:645, 1953.

274. BRICK, I. B.: Clinical significance of aminoaciduria. *New England J. Med., 247*:635, 1952.

275. UZMAN, L. L., IBER, F. L., CHALMERS, T. C., and KNOWLTON, M.: The mechanism of copper deposition in the liver in hepatolenticular degeneration (Wilson's disease). *Am. J. M. Sc., 231*:511, 1956.

276. STEIN, W. H., BEARN, A. G., and MOORE, S.: The aminoacid content of the blood and urine in Wilson's disease. *J. Clin. Investigation, 33*:410, 1954.

277. WARNOCK, C. G., and NEILL, D. W.: Dimercaprol in the pre-neurological stage of Wilson's disease (hepatolenticular degeneration). *J. Neurol. Neurosurg. & Psychiat., 17*:70, 1954.

278. BOUDIN, G., PEPIN, B., and CALATCHI, R.: Cas familial de degenerescence hepato-lenticulaire troubles du metabolisme des acides amines et du cuivre. Effets du traitment par le B.A.L. *Rev. neurol., 87*:271, 1952.

279. BEARN, A. G., and KUNKEL, H. G.: Abnormalities of copper metabolism in Wilson's disease and their relationship to the aminoaciduria. *J. Clin. Investigation. 33*:400, 1954.

280. BEARN, A. G.: Genetic and biochemical aspects of Wilson's disease. *Am. J. Med., 15*:442, 1953.

281. ANDRE, M. J., and VAN BOGAERT, L.: L'heredite dans la degenerescence hepato-lenticulaire et le probleme des rapports intrinseques de la pseudosclerose de Westphal-Strumpell et de la maladie de Wilson. *L'Encephale, 39*:1, 1950.

282. STADLER, H.: Histopathologische Untersuchungen zur Frage der Beziehung Zwischen Leber-und-Gehirnveranderungen. *Ztschr. ges. Neurol. u. Psychiat., 154*:626, 1935.

283. Coke, L. R., and Shaw, E. G.: Hepato-lenticular degeneration. *Canad. M. A. J.,* 73:967, 1955.

284. Cohen, I. M.: Recent advances in the therapy of hepatolenticular degeneration. *Dis. Nerv. System,* 14:95, 1953.

285. Walshe, J. M.: Wilson's disease, new oral therapy. *Lancet,* 270:25, 1956.

286. Walshe, J. M.: Penicillamine, a new oral therapy for Wilson's disease. *Am. J. Med.,* 21:487, 1956.

287. Ostertog, B.: Uber eine Neuartige Heredogenerative Erkrankungs Form Lokaliziert im Striatum und Rinde mit Ansegedehnter Myelolyse. *Arch. Psychiat.,* 77:354, 1926.

288. von Braunmuhl, A.: Die Rinden Markkomponente im Anatomischen Bild der Wilson-Pseudosklerose Grupp. *Ztxchr. ges. Neurol. u. Psychiat.,* 130:1, 1930.

289. Richter, R.: The pallial component in hepatolenticular degeneration. *J. Neuropath. & Exper. Neurol.,* 7:1, 1948.

290. Jervis, G. A., Notkin, J., Freiman, I. S., and Moore, J.: Progressive lenticular degeneration. *Psychiat. Quart.,* 16:369, 1942.

291. Scherer, H. J.: Zur Frage der Beziehung Zwischen Leber und Gehirnverandergungen. *Virchows Arch.,* 288:333, 1933.

292. Adams, R. O., and Davidson, C.: Discussants on Paper—The central nervous system in hepatic disease. *J. Neuropath. & Exper. Neurol.,* 8:283, 1949.

293. Alexander, L.: The fundamental type of histopathological changes encountered in cases of athetosis and paralysis agitous. *A. Res. Nerv. & Ment. Dis. Proc.,* 21:334, 1942.

294. Neppi, A.: Sulle Alterazioni Cadaverich delle Cellule Nervese Rilevabili col Metado de Nissl. *Riv. pat. nerv.,* Firenze, 2:152, 1897.

295. Barbacci, O., and Campacci, G.: Sulle Lesioni Cadaveriche delle cellule Nervose. *Riv. pat. nerv.,* Firenze, 2:227, 1897.

296. Koenig, R. S., and Koenig, H.: An experimental study of postmortem alterations in neurons of the central nervous system. *J. Neuropath. & Exper. Neurol.,* 11:69, 1952.

297. Jungmann, H., and Kimmelstiel, P.: Uber den Ursprung der Milchsoure im Zentralnervensystem. *Biochem. Ztschr.,* 212:347, 1929.

298. Weil, A.: *Textbook of Neuropathology,* 2nd Ed. New York, Grune & Stratton, 1945.

299. Quastel, J. H., and Wheatley, A. H. M.: Oxidations by the brain, *Biochem.,* 26:725, 1932.

300. Wilens, L.: The relationship of chronic alcoholism to atherosclerosis. *J.A.M.A.,* 135:1136, 1947.

301. Weil, A.: The influence of formolin fixation on the lipids of the central nervous system. *J. Biol. Chem.,* 83:601, 1929.

302. Inose, T.: Hepatocerebral degeneration, a special type. *J. Neuropath. & Exper. Neurol.,* 11:40, 1952.

303. Statler, H.: Weitere Untersuchungen zum Wilson-Pseudosklerose-Problem, *Ztschr. ges. Neurol. u. Psychiat.,* 158:92, 1937.

304. Konowolow, N. W.: Uber eigenartige Veranderungen der Nervenzellen bei Hepatolenticularer Degeneration und Underen Hepatocerebralen Erkrankungen. *Ztschr. ges Neurol. u. psychiat.,* 171:229, 1941.

305. WOOD, A. H., and PENDELTON, L.: Fourteen simultaneous cases of an acute degenerative striatal disease. *Arch. Neurol. & Psychiat., 13*:549, 1925.
306. SIEMERLING, E., and JACOB, A.: Klinischer und Anatomischer Beitrog zur Lehre von der Pseudosklerose Westphal-Strümpell mit Coronea Ring und Doppelseitiger Scheinkatarakt. *Deutsche Ztschr. Nervenh.*, p. 123, 1932.
307. SCHMIDT, M.: Etudes sur la pathogenese de la degeneriscence hepato-Lenticulaire. *Acta psychiat. et Neurol., 5*:163, 1930.
308. KORNYEY, S.: Zur Nosographie und Histopathologie der Striaren Erkrankungen Degeneration Natur. *Deutsche Ztschr. Nervenh., 108*:39, 1929.
309. TSCHUNGUNOFF, S. A.: Zur Frage der Pathologischen Anatomie und Pathogenese der Wilsonschen Krankheit. *Ztschr. ges. Neurol. u. Psychiat., 86*: 506, 1923.
310. SCHARENBERG, K., and BROWN, E. D.: Histopathology of catatonic states. A study with silver carbonate. *J. Neuropath. & Exper. Neurol., 13*:592, 1954.
311. PAGE, I. H.: *Chemistry of the Brain.* Springfield, Thomas, 1937.
312. ELLIOTT, K. A. C., PAGE, I. H., and QUASTEL, J. H.: *Neurochemistry.* Springfield, Thomas, 1955.
313. WOOLLAM, D. H. M., and MILLEN, J. W.: The morphology of the blood brain barrier. IInd International Congress of Neuropathology, London 1955.
314. McINTOSH, J. E., FRENCH, L. A., PEYTON, W. T., and GRUNDLAND, B.: Studies on cerebrovascular permeability. *Bull. Univ. Minnesota Hosp., 28*:250, 1957.
315. BROMAN, T., and LINDBERG-BROMAN, A. M.: An experimental study of disorders in the permeability of the cerebral vessels (the blood) brain barrier) produced by clinical and physiochemical agents. *Acta physiol. scandinav., 10*:102, 1945.
316. BAKAY, L.: Discussion: Weekly clinicopathological exercises case records of the Massachusetts General Hosp. *New England J. Med., 251*:617, 1954.
317. BAKAY, L.: *The Blood-Brain Barrier.* Springfield, Thomas, 1956.
318. COHN, P., GAITONDE, M. K., and RICHTER, D.: The uptake into the rat brain of S^{35} methionine administered by different routes. Neuropsych. Res. Centre Whitechurch Hosp. Cardiff 1955.
319. KETY, S.: Blood flow and metabolism of the human brain in health and disease, in *Neurochemistry* by Elliott, K. A. C., Page, I. H., Quastel, J. H. Springfield, Thomas, 1955 p. 302.
320. FAZEKAS, J. F., TICKTIN, H. E., EHRMANTRAUT, W. R., and ALMAN, R. W.: Cerebral metabolism in hepatic insufficiency. *Am. J. Med., 21*:843, 1956.
321. EISENMENGER, W. J., BLONDHEIM, S. H., BONGIOVAUNI, A. M., and KUNKEL, H. G.: Electrolyte studies on patients with cirrhosis of the liver. *J. Clin. Investigation, 29*:1491, Nov. 1950.
322. KUNKEL, H. G.: Factors in the mechanism of ascites. in *Liver Disease,* Ciba Symposium, Philadelphia, Blakiston, 1951, p. 130.
323. CHALMERS, T. C.: Discussion: Studies on "alcoholic" cirrhosis and chronic recurrent fluid retention and ascites, in *Liver Disease,* Ciba, Symposium, Philadelphia, Blakiston, 1951, p. 162.

324. MARK, R. M.: Discussion: Factors in the Production of Ascites, in *Liver Disease*, Ciba Symposium, Philadelphia, Blakiston, 1951, p. 168.

325. IVERSEN, P.: The pathogenesis of ascites, in *Liver Disease*, Ciba Symposium, Philadelphia, Blakiston, 1951, p. 136.

326. AMATUZIO, D. S., STUTZMAN, F., SHRIFTER, N., and NESBITT, S.: A study of serum electrolytes in patients with severely decompensated portal cirrhosis of the liver. *J. Lab. & Clin. Med., 39*:26, 1952.

327. VANAMEE, P., POPPELL, J. W., GLICKSMAN, A. S., RANDALL, H. T., and ROBERTS, K. E.: *Respiratory alkalosis in hepatic coma. Arch. Int. Med., 97*:762, 1956.

328. CARRYA, H. M.: Tissue anoxia resulting from respiratory alkalosis, *Proc. Staff Meet., Mayo Clin., 22*:456, 1947.

329. DARROW, C. W., and PATHMAN, J. H.: Relation of heart rate to slow waves in the electroencephalogram during over ventilation. *Am. J. Physiol., 140*:583, 1944.

330. FEIGIN, I., and WOLF, A.: The phosphatases of the nervous system. *J. Neuropath. & Exper. Neurol., 14*:11, 1955.

331. ROIZIN, L.: Oxidases and peroxidases of the central nervous system. *J. Neuropath. & Exper. Neural., 14*:47, 1955.

332. HOLMBERG, C. G., and LAURELL, C. B.: Investigation in serum copper. Part I. Nature of serum copper and its relation to iron-binding protein in human serum. *Acta chem. scandinav., 1*:944, 1947.

333. HOLMBERG, C. G., and LAURELL, C. B.: Investigations in serum copper. Part II. Isolation of the copper containing protein, and a description of some of its properties, *Acta chem. scandinav., 2*:550, 1948.

334. GUBLER, C. J.: Copper metabolism in man. *J.A.M.A., 161*:530, 1956.

335. VAN RAVESTYN, A. H.: Metabolism of copper in urine. *Acta med. scandinav. 118*:163, 1944.

336. BENNETTS, H. W., and CHAPMAN, F. E.: Copper deficiency in sheep in Western Australia; a preliminary account of the etiology of enzootic ataxia of lambs and of anemia of ewes. *Australian Vet. J., 13*:138, 1937.

337. DUNLOP, G., INNES, J. R. M., SHEARER, G. D., and WELLS, H. E.: Swayback studies in North Derbyshire. *J. Am. Path. & Therapeutics, 52*:259, 1939.

338. BENNETTS, H. W., and BECK, A. B.: Enzootic ataxia and copper deficiency of sheep in Western Australia. *Bull. Counc. Sci. Indust. Res. Australia*, No. 147, 1942.

339. CAMPBELL, A. M. G., DANIEL, P., PORTER, R. J., RUSSELL, W. R. R., SMITH, H., and INNES, J. R. M.: Disease of the nervous system occurring among research workers on swayback in lambs. *Brain, 70*:50, 1947.

340. TINGEY, A. H.: The iron, copper and manganese content of the human brain. *J. Ment. Sc., 83*:452, 1937.

341. KLUVER, H.: Porphyrins, the nervous system, and behaviour. *J. Psychol., 17*:209, 1944.

342. ELEVEHJEM, C. A.: The biological significance of copper and its relation to iron metabolism. *Physiol. Rev., 15*:471, 1935.

343. KIEL, H. L., and NELSON, V. W.: The role of copper in carbohydrate metabolism. *J. Biol. Chem., 106*:343, 1934.

344. FLESCH, P.: The role of Cu in mammalian pigmentation. *Proc. Soc. Exper. Biol. & Med.,* 70:79, 1949.

345. CARTWRIGHT, G. E.: Copper metabolism in human subjects, symposium, *Animal and Soil Relationship,* Johns Hopkins Univ., McCollum-Pratt Inst., W. D. McElroy Ed., 1950, p. 274.

346. MARBLE, A., and SMITH, M.: Studies of iron metabolism in a case of hemochromatosis. *Ann. Int. Med.,* 12:1592, 1939.

347. BENDA, L., and RISSEL, E.: Iron metabolism in acute diseases of parenchyma. *Wien. Klin. Wchnschr.,* 61:816-818, Nov. 25, 1949.

348. SHELDEN, J. H.: Hemochromatosis. *Lancet,* 2:1031, 1934.

349. GRANICK, S.: Iron metabolism and hemochromatosis. *Bull. New York Acad. Med.,* 25:403-428, 1949.

350. LUCIANO, A.: Iron metabolism in hemochromatosis. *Rassegna Fisiopat. clin. e terap.,* 21:279, 1949.

351. BELSASSO, E., and ZUCONI, V.: Studies on the iron metabolism in liver patients. II Chronic diseases of the liver. *Riv. gastroenterol.,* 2:219, 1951.

352. GITLOW, S. E., and BEYERS, M. R.: Metabolism of iron I. Intravenous tolerance tests in normal subjects and patients with hemochromatosis, *J. Lab. & Clin. Med.,* 39:337, 1952.

353. VOLLAND, W.: Iron and copper metabolism of brain. *Med. Monatsschr.,* 3:246-253, April 1949.

354. SHELDEN, J. H.: The iron content of the tissues in hemochromatosis with special reference to the brain. *Quart. J. Med.,* 21:123, 1927.

355. HOWARD, R. B.: The serum iron in diseases of the liver. *J. Clin. Investigation,* 29:824, 1950.

356. GILLMAN, J., MANDELSTAM, J., and GILMAN, T.: Comparison of chemical and histologic estimations of iron and copper contents of Africans in relation to the pathogenesis of cytosiderosis and cirrhosis (hemochromatosis). *South African J. M. Sc.,* 10:109, 1945.

357. VANOTTI, A., and DELACHAUX, A.: *Iron Metabolism and Its Clinical Significance.* London, Muller, 1949.

358. FRANDSEN, S.: On the metabolism of iron in hemochromatosis. *Acta med. scandinav.,* 128:186, 1947.

359. CARTWRIGHT, G. E.: Dietary factors concerned in erythropoeisis, *Blood,* 2:256, 1947.

360. WARBURG, O., and CHRISTIAN, W.: *Uber die Katalytischen Wirkungen der Lebendigen Substanz.* Berlin, J. Springer, 1928.

361. WARBURG, O., and CHRISTIAN, W.: Uber Aktivierung der Robinsonchen Hexose-Mona-Phosphorsaure in Roten Blutzellen und die Gewinnung Aktinierender Fermenltosungen. *Biochem. Ztschr.,* 242:206, 1931.

362. WARBURG, O., and CHRISTIAN, W.: Uber ein Neues Oxydationsferment und Sein Absorptionsspektrum, *Biochem. Ztschr.,* 254:438, 1932.

363. WARBURG, O., and CHRISTIAN, W.: Verbrennung von Robison-Ester durch Triphospho-Pyridin-Nucleotid. *Biochem. Ztschr.,* 287:440, 1936.

364. KEILIN, D., and HARTREE, E. F.: Prosthetic group of glucose oxidase. *Nature,* 157:801, 1946.

365. KEILIN, D., and HARTREE, E. F.: Properties of glucose oxidase. *Biochem. J.,* 42:221, 1948.

366. HIMWICH, H. E.: *Brain Metabolism and Cerebral Disorders.* Baltimore Williams & Wilkins, 1951.

367. EMBDEN, G., DENTICKE, H. J., and KRAFT, G.: Uber die Intermediaren Vargange bei der Glykolyse in der Muskulatur. *Klin. Wchnschr., 12*:213, 1933.

368. MEYERHOF, O.: Oxidoreductions in carbohydrate breakdown. *Biol. Symposia, 5*:141, 1941.

369. CORI, C. F.: The kinetics of the enzymatic synthesis of glycogen from clucose-1-phosphate. *J. Biol. Chem., 135*:733, 1940.

370. KEILIN, D.: On cytochrome, a respiratory pigment, common to animals, yeast and higher plants. *Proc. Roy. Soc., London, 98*:312, 1925.

371. KEILIN, D.: Cytochrome and respiratory enzymes. *Proc. Roy. Soc., London, 104*:206, 1928.

372. LEMBERG, R., and LEGGE, J. W.: *Hematin Compounds and Bile Pigments.* New York, Interscience, 1949.

373. SPATZ, H.: Uber den Eisennachweis im Gehirn Besonders in den Zentren des Extropyramidal Motorischen Systems. *Ztschr. ges. Neurol. u. Psychiat., 77*:261, 1922.

374. FERRONI, A.: Recent data on iron metabolism in extra pyramidal affections. *Acta neurol.,* Napoli, *5*:419, 1950.

375. NAPIER, L. E.: A case of iron encephalopathy. *Indian M. Gaz., 71*:143, 1936.

376. BIRCH, C. A., and HILL, M.: Iron encephalopathy. *Brit. M. J., 4697*:62, Jan. 13, 1951.

377. PETERSON, R. E.: The serum iron in acute hepatitis. *J. Lab. & Clin. Med., 39*:1, 225, 1952.

378. KIPPING, H., and SCHMOLDT, H.: The importance of iron in diseases of the liver. *Deutsch. Arch. Klin. Med., 198*:434, 1951.

379. STRASSMANN, G.: Iron and calcium deposits in the brain and their pathologic significance. *J. Neuropath. & Exper. Neurol., 8*:8, 1949.

380. STRASSMANN, G.: Hemosiderin and tissue iron: Relationship occurrences and importance; study on 93 human brains. *J. Neuropath. & Exper. Neurol., 4*:393, Oct. 1945.

381. NEUMAN, M.: Hemochromatosis of the central nervous system. *J. Neuropath. & Exper. Neurol, 7*:19, 1948.

382. WISLOCKI, G. B., and PUTNAM, T. J.: Further observation on the anatomy and physiology of the area postrema. *Anat. Rec., 27*:151, 1924.

383. KRAININ, P., and KAHN, B. S.: Hemochromatosis: Report of a case in a Negro; Discussion of iron metabolism. *Ann. Int. Med., 33*:453, 1950.

384. HERBUT, P. A., WATSON, J. S., and PERKINS, E.: Alloxan in experimental hemochromatosis. *Am. J. Clin. Path., 16*:506, 1946.

385. MANN, F. C.: The effects of complete and partial removal of the liver. *Medicine, 6*:419, 1927.

386. VAN SLYKE, D. D., and MEYER, G. M.: The fate of protein digestion products in the body. *J. Biol. Chem., 16*:213, 1913.

387. BOLLMANN, J. L., MANN, F. C., and MAGATH, T. B.: Studies on the physiology of the liver. *Am. J. Physiol., 69*:371, 1924.

388. BLASS, J., COCHIN, M., and DURLACH, J.: Use of micro-paper chromatography in the study of aminoaciduria, in cirrhosis; continuous presence of tyrosine in the sea of cirrhosis. *Bull. et mém Soc. méd. Hôp., Paris,* 66:1253, 1950.

389. SCHREIER, K.: Investigations on amino acid metabolism and hepatic diseases. *Deutsche med. Wchnschr.,* 76:26, 868-872, June 29, 1951.

390. GREENE, C. H.: Liver and biliary tract: Review for 1940. *Arch. Int. Med.,* 67:867-888, 1941.

391. EARLE, D. P., and VICTOR, J.: The effects of various diets on the liver damage caused by excess cystine. *J. Exper. Med.,* 75:179, 1942.

392. MOREHEAD, R. P., FISHMAN, W. H., and ARTOM, C.: Renal injury in the rat following the administration of serine by stomach tube. *Am. J. Path.,* 21:803, 1945.

393. SCHWERIN, P., BASSMAN, S. P., and WAELSCH, H.: The uptake of glutamic acid and glutamine by brain and other tissues of the rat and mouse. *J. Biol. Chem.,* 184:37, 1950.

394. BOULANGER, P.: Glutamic acid and cerebral metabolism. *Exposes Ann. Biochem. Med.,* Paris Series, 13:119, 1951.

395. KREBS, H. A.: Metabolism of amino acids, IV the synthesis of glutamine from glutamic acid and ammonia, and the enzymic hydrolysis of glutamine in animal tissues. *J. Biol. Chem.,* 29:2, 1951, 1935.

396. MAYER-GROSS, W., and WALKER, J. W.: The effect of 1. Glutamic acid and other amino acids in hypoglycemia. *Biochem. J.,* 44:92, 1949.

397. BOREK, E., MILLER, H. K., SHEINESS, P., and WAELSCH, H.: The effect of the sulfoxide from dl-methionine on glutamic acid and glutamine metabolism. *J. Biol. Chem.,* 163:347, 1946.

398. WAELSCH, H., OWADES, P., MILLER, A. K., and BOREK, E.: Glutamic acid anti-metabolites sulfonide derived from methionine. *J. Biol. Chem.,* 166:273, 1946.

399. BONDY, P. K.: Glucose metabolic defects in hepatic diseases, Am. Assoc. Liver Dis., Chicago, Ill. Nov. 3, 1955. *Lancet,* 269:1322, 1955.

400. MEYERHOF, O.: *Carbohydrate Metabolism in Brain Tissue, The Biology of Mental Health and Disease.* New York, Hoeber, 1952, p. 84.

401. WILLIAMS, R. H., and BISSELL, G. W.: Thiamine metabolism with particular reference to the role of the liver and kidneys. *Arch. Int. Med.,* 73:203, 1944.

402. PETERS, R. A.: The biochemical lesion in vitamin B_1 deficiency. *Lancet,* 230:1161, 1936.

403. GEIGER, A., MAGNES, J., TAYLOR, R. M., and VERALLI, M.: Effect of blood constituents on uptake of glucose and on metabolic rate of the brain in perfusion experiments. *Am. J. Physiol.,* 177:138, 1954.

404. BAKER, A. B., and WATSON, C. J.: Central nervous system in porphyria. *J. Neuropath. & Exper. Neurol.,* 4:1945.

405. POTTER, V. R., and DUBOIS, K. P.: The quantitative determination of cytochrome C. *J. Biol. Chem.,* 142:417, 1942.

406. SCHWARTZ, S.: Personal communication.

407. WARBURG, O.: Uber die Wirkung von Kohlenoxyd und Stickoxyd auf Atmung und Garung. *Biochem. Ztschr.,* 189:354, 1927.

408. JOHNSON, A. J., McNABB, A. R., and ROSSITER, R. J.: Concentration of lipids in the brain of infants and adults. *Biochem. J.*, 44:494, 1949.

409. TYRRELL, L. W., and RICHTER, D.: The lipids of cell nuclei isolated from human brain cortex. *Biochem. J.*, London, 49:51, 1951.

410. GEYER, R. P., MATHEW, L. W., and STARE, F. J.: Metabolism of emulsified trilourin (-C 1400-) and octanoic acid (-C 1400-) by rat tissue slices, *J. Biol. Chem.*, 180:1037, 1949.

411. SPERRY, W. M.: *Lipid Metabolism of the Brain, The Biology of Mental Health and Disease.* New York, Hoeber, 1952, p. 116.

412. FISK, A., Chanutin, A., and KLINGMAN, W. D.: Lipids and proteins of plasma in patients with diseases of the nervous system. *Arch. Neurol & Psychiat.*, 67:332, 1952.

413. CRANDALL, L. A., and CHERRY, I. S.: Blood lipase, diastase, and esterase in M. S. *Arch. Neurol. & Psychiat.*, 27:373, 1932.

414. WEIL, A., and CLEVELAND, D. A.: A serologic study of M. S. *Arch. Neurol. & Psychiat.*, 27:375, 1932.

415. GIGLI, G.: Lipaemia in hepatocellular jaundice. *Riv. gastroenterol.*, Parma, 1:137, 1949.

416. CORNATZER, W. E., and CAYER, D.: Phospholipid synthesis in patients with cirrhosis and infectious hepatitis. *South. M. J.*, 43:212, 1950.

417. NOVA, G.: The effect of lipotropic factors on phospholipids and cerebrosides in the blood of patients with liver cirrhosis. *Rassegna fisiopat. clin. e terap.*, 21:764, 1949.

418. MAN, E. B., KARTIN, B. L., DURLACHER, S. H., and PETERS, J. P.: The lipids of serum and liver in patients with hepatic diseases. *J. Clin. Investigation*, 24:623, 1945.

419. PIERCE, F. T., and GOFMAN, J. W.: Lipoproteins, liver disease and atherosclerosis. *Circulation*, 4:25, 1951.

420. JERVIS, G. A.: Occurrence of brain hemorrhages in choline deficient rats. *Proc. Soc. Exper. Biol. & Med.*, 51:193, 1942.

421. FOA, B. P., WEINSTEIN, H. R., and KLEPPEL, B.: Lipids of rat brain and liver in choline deficiency. *Arch. Biochem.*, 19:209, 1948.

422. HURST, E. W.: Experimental demyelination of the central nervous system. *J. Exper. Biol. & M. Sc.*, 20:297, 1942.

423. BAKER, A. B.: Central nervous system in tetanus. *J. Neuropath. & Exper. Neurol.*, 1:394, 1942.

424. RIVERS, T. M., and SCHWENTKER, F. F.: Encephalitis accompanied by myelin destruction. *J. Exper. Med.*, 61:689, 1935.

425. FERRARO, A.: Experimental toxic encephalomyelopathy, diffuse sclerosis following subcutaneous injections of potassium cyanide. *Arch. Neurol. & Psychiat.*, 29:1364, 1933.

426. WEIL, A.: The effect of hemolytic toxins on nervous tissue. *Arch. Path.*, 9:828, 1930.

427. SPERRY, W. M., and WAELSCH, H.: The chemistry of myelination and demyelination. *A. Res. Nerv. & Ment. Dis., Proc.*, 28:255, 1950.

428. OCHOA, S.: *Pyruvate Oxidation in the Brain, The Biology of Mental Health and Disease.* New York, Hoeber, 1951, p. 97.

429. DUTLIN, W. B.: Pathogenesis of kernicterus. *J. Neuropath. & Exper. Neurol.*, 8:119, 1949.

430. JOHNSON, B. B., and LUETSCHER, J. A.: The possible role of aldosterone in edema. *Ann. New York Acad. Sc., 61*:605, 1955.

431. GYORGY, P.: Effects of antibiotics and vitamin B₁₂ in cirrhosis and necrosis of the liver, in *Liver Disease*, Ciba Symposium. Philadelphia, Blakiston, 1951, p. 81.

432. EINARSON, L.: Notes on the histochemical aspect of the changes of the spinal motot cells in anoxia, vitamin E deficiency and poliomyelitis. *Acta orthop. Scandinav., 19*:55, 1950.

433. EINARSON, L.: Criticizing review of the concepts of the neuromuscular lesions in experimental vit. E deficiency preferably in adult rats. *Acta Psychiat. et Neurol., Suppl.* 78, 1952.

434. VALLEE, B. L., WACKER, W. E. C., BARTHOLOMAY, K. F., and ROBIN, E. B.: Serum zinc concentrations in Laennec's cirrhosis and their validation by sequential analysis. *New England J. Med., 225*:403, 1956.

435. VALLEE, B. L.: The metabolic role of zinc. *J. A. M. A., 162*:1053, 1956.

436. CAREY, J. B.: The serum dihydroxy-trihydroxy bile acid ratio in liver and biliary tract disease. *J. Clin. Invest., 35*:695, 1956.

437. HOCKENHULL, D.: Inhibition of a succini aerodehydrogenase system by surface-active agents. *Nature, 162*:850, 1948.

438. ASHMORE, J., and NESBETT, F. B.: Effect of bile acids on activity of glucose -6- phosphatase. *Proc. Soc. Exper. Biol. & Med., 89*:78, 1955.

439. MANN, E.: Action of bile and bile salts on the adenosine-triphosphatase (ATPase) activity of myosin. *Arch. sc. biol.* 38:295, 1954.

440. TAKATA, H.: Über den Einfluss der Gallensaure auf Glycerophosphotase. *J. Biochem., 14*:61, 1931.

441. EICHEL, B., WAINIO, W. W., and PERSON, P.: A partial separation and characterization of cytochrome oxidase and cytochrome -b. *J. Biol. chem., 183*:89, 1950.

442. McCORMICK, H. M., and DRILL, V. A.: Lipotropic effects of liver extract, vitamin B₁₂ and choline. *Proc. Soc. Exper. Biol. & Med., 74*:626, 1950.

443. ALEXANDER, W. F., and BACKLAR, B.: Nucleic acid changes in rat nerve tissue after parenteral administration of vitamin B₁₂. *Proc. Soc. Exper. Biol. & Med.,* 78:181, 1951.

444. JONES, P. N., and MILLS, E. H.: The effect of liver disease on serum vitamin B₁₂ concentrations. *J. Clin. Investigation, 35*:717, 1956.

445. SHERLOCK, S.: *Discussion: Circulatory studies on patients with ascites, in Liver Disease,* Ciba Symposium. Philadelphia, Blakiston, 1951, p. 182.